BOTTOM LINE'S
RED FLAGS

TABLE OF CONTENTS

BOTTOM LINE'S RED FLAGS

COMMON SYMPTOMS NEVER TO IGNORE

Source: **J. Edward Hill, MD,** president-elect of the American Medical Association and an editor of *American Medical Association Family Medical Guide*. Wiley. He is a family physician at North Mississippi Medical Center and a faculty member at Family Medicine Residency Center, both in Tupelo.

Symptoms we all experience occasionally, such as upset stomach or headache, rarely are cause for concern. Yet even mild symptoms may be a sign of serious underlying illness. The challenge is knowing when you can treat yourself and when you need medical attention.

Common symptoms—and when they may be dangerous...

ABDOMINAL PAIN...

This is one of the most difficult symptoms to evaluate because it can be caused by hundreds of conditions.

USUAL CAUSES: Gas, stress, viral or bacterial infections (such as food poisoning).

WARNING: Abdominal pain that lasts more than a day or two ...causes severe cramps...or is accompanied by other symptoms, such as persistent nausea or vomiting, should be evaluated by a physician. **THE PROBLEM COULD BE...**

• *Appendicitis.* Patients often experience fever or nausea as well as intense stomach pain. The pain typically begins around the navel and shifts to the lower-right abdomen over six to 12 hours. If the appendix isn't surgically removed before it ruptures, it can cause a life-threatening infection called peritonitis.

• *Gallbladder disease, gallstones, ulcers and stomach cancer* can cause abdominal pain ranging from sharp and intermittent to dull and constant.

BACK PAIN...

Back pain is a leading cause of lost workdays. Even minor back injuries can cause excruciating pain.

USUAL CAUSES: Muscle pulls or spasms cause 90% of back pain. Apply an ice pack as often as possible during the first 24 hours after pain starts...switch to heat after 24 hours...and take a nonsteroidal anti-inflammatory drug, such as aspirin or ibuprofen, to control pain and swelling.

If back pain does not improve after a week, see your doctor.

WARNING: Back pain that is accompanied by fever and neurological symptoms, such as tingling, numbness or shooting pains down one or both legs, is potentially serious. These symptoms may indicate a spinal infection, which is relatively rare but can cause permanent damage. See your doctor or go to an emergency room immediately.

CHEST PAIN...

Any pain in the chest should be taken seriously because it is a common symptom of heart attack.

USUAL CAUSE: Musculoskeletal injury caused by overexertion. Working all day in the yard or pushing too hard at the gym can result in a muscle pull between the ribs or in the upper chest. This may cause a dull ache or shooting pains.

If pain occurs only when you move your body in a certain way, it is probably caused by a strained muscle or inflammation in the ribs (costochondritis). The pain usually subsides in a day or two.

WARNING: Suspect a heart attack if the pain is accompanied by a pressing or crushing sensation, radiates out from the chest to other parts of the body (such as the breastbone, jaw, arms or neck) and/or is accompanied by heavy sweating, nausea or vomiting. Call 911 immediately. Then take an aspirin, unlock your door and wait for help to arrive.

Severe chest pain that occurs in patients who recently have had surgery or been bedridden due to illness or injury may be caused by a pulmonary embolism (blood clot in the lung). Again, get medical assistance immediately.

CONSTIPATION...

The frequency of bowel movements is highly variable—from twice a day to several times a week may be normal. Any change in your usual habits deserves attention.

USUAL CAUSES: Most constipation is due to insufficient fiber and/or water in the diet. Try to get at least 25 grams of fiber daily. Start the day with a high-fiber cereal, such as oatmeal... snack on fresh fruits...and eat more beans, whole grains and vegetables. Drink two quarts of liquid daily (water is best).

Also, exercise for at least 20 minutes most days of the week. Exercise stimulates intestinal contractions that promote bowel movements.

WARNING: Sudden constipation or alternating bouts of diarrhea and constipation may be a sign of colon cancer. Call your doctor—you may need a colonoscopy to determine if cancer is present.

FATIGUE...

It's normal to be exhausted after a hard day, but persistent fatigue isn't normal, especially when it suddenly worsens.

USUAL CAUSES: A combination of inadequate sleep and bad diet, such as loading up on coffee or junk food, can cause fatigue. Caffeine is a stimulant—but after the initial stimulation, people often experience "rebound fatigue." Junk food usually is high in carbohydrates, which can cause a surge in blood sugar followed by a drop, resulting in fatigue.

Limit your intake of caffeinated beverages to one or two servings daily. Go to bed and get up at the same times most days of the week. Eat nutritious meals, and exercise regularly —it promotes deeper sleep.

WARNING: Fatigue can be a symptom of almost all diseases, but people who experience more fatigue than usual—in the absence of any lifestyle changes—should get an immediate checkup.

HEADACHE...

Anyone who gets headaches more than once a month or is incapacitated by a headache needs to get a complete medical workup immediately.

USUAL CAUSES: About 90% of headaches are tension headaches, caused by fatigue or emotional stress. Aspirin, ibuprofen and acetaminophen are effective at relieving pain—see which works best for you. Stress-reduction techniques, such as yoga, also can help.

Migraine headaches are more severe, but they usually can be controlled or prevented with ibuprofen or prescription drugs, such as *sumatriptan* (Imitrex).

WARNING: Headaches that increase in frequency...are unusually severe...or are accompanied by other symptoms, such as nausea, slurred speech or vision changes, should be brought to a doctor's attention immediately. They could be a sign of stroke, infection in a brain blood vessel, meningitis or even a brain tumor.

IMPORTANT: Call 911 if you suspect a stroke or experience an excruciating headache that comes out of the blue. This is know as a "thunderclap" headache, and it may be due to a potentially fatal ruptured blood vessel in the brain.

HEARTBURN...

Most of us have experienced this burning sensation behind the breastbone.

USUAL CAUSE: Indigestion, often from eating fatty or spicy foods.

WARNING: Gastroesophageal reflux disease (GERD) is a common cause of heartburn. Mild cases can be treated with antacids, but GERD that occurs more than once a week can cause serious damage to the esophagus. There's also a link between chronic GERD and esophageal cancer. Patients usually require acid-blocking medications, such as *omeprazole* (Prilosec) or *ranitidine* (Zantac).

HELPFUL: If you need antacids more than once or twice a week, see your doctor.

■

WHAT YOU REALLY NEED TO KNOW ABOUT PREVENTING CANCER

Source: **Richard S. Rivlin, MD**, professor of medicine, Weill Medical College of Cornell University and director, Anne Fisher Nutrition Center at Strang Cancer Prevention Center, both in New York City. He is also a consultant at Memorial Sloan-Kettering Cancer Center, New York City.

Cancer claims the lives of 1,500 Americans each day, but up to two-thirds of these malignancies could be prevented.

Millions of Americans have taken cancer prevention to heart and made lifestyle changes—eating a nutritious diet, maintaining a healthful weight and not smoking.

now: The latest cancer research has identified other important prevention strategies that most people don't take seriously enough.

Key mistakes that you should avoid...

1. *Inhaling secondhand smoke.* Each year, tobacco use causes approximately 180,000 cancer deaths. Millions of Americans have quit smoking, but most people underestimate the risk of even occasional exposure to secondhand smoke.

The Environmental Protection Agency (EPA) estimates that secondhand smoke causes approximately 3,000 cases of lung cancer in the US annually. If you live with someone who smokes, your risk of dying from lung cancer is 30% higher than if you live in a smoke-free environment.

SELF-DEFENSE: Avoid secondhand smoke by asking guests to smoke outside, for example, or staying away from groups of smokers outside office buildings. This will immediately reduce your risk of developing cancers of the lung, throat, bladder, kidney, pancreas and mouth.

BONUS: A study published in the *British Medical Journal* reported that hospital admissions for heart attacks dropped by 60% in Helena, Montana, when the city adopted a smoke-free policy. As little as 30 minutes of exposure to secondhand smoke is hazardous to people with heart or lung conditions.

2. *Not getting annual skin exams.* There are approximately 1 million cases of non-melanoma skin cancer diagnosed annually in the US—plus more than 54,000 Americans are diagnosed with melanoma, the deadliest skin cancer. Melanoma is

15 to 20 times more common now than it was 50 years ago, in part because of depletion of the ozone layer.

Skin cancer is among the most preventable and easily treated of all cancers, yet few doctors perform full skin exams during routine checkups. Insist on it. The vast majority of melanomas can be cured if they're detected and treated at an early stage.

SELF-DEFENSE: At least once a year, ask your primary-care physician or dermatologist to check your entire body for changes in the size or color of moles or other darkly pigmented areas and/or new growths. Make sure your doctor examines areas that are often missed, such as the scalp, soles of the feet and genitals.

SMART IDEA: Ask your doctor to take photographs of suspicious spots to watch. The pictures will provide a baseline comparison for future checkups.

3. *Settling for sigmoidoscopy.* Colon cancer also is among the most treatable of cancers when it's detected early, yet nearly 48,000 Americans die from it needlessly each year.

Unfortunately, many doctors still continue to recommend flexible sigmoidoscopy as the only necessary procedure. This test—in which a lighted, hollow tube is inserted through the rectum—views only the lower half of the colon. Cancers or precancerous polyps present in the upper half of the colon are missed entirely by the procedure.

Colonoscopy is a better choice because it views the entire colon. A study that compared the two tests found that nearly half of 128 patients with advanced cancers or *adenomas* (abnormal growths that can develop into cancer) had them in the upper colon only—the area not examined by sigmoidoscopy.

SELF-DEFENSE: Get a colonoscopy every 10 years, starting at age 50. Patients with risk factors (a family history of colon cancer or a diagnosis of inflammatory bowel disease) may be advised to start getting the test as early as age 35 or 40.

4. *Cutting good dietary fat.* Most Americans have reduced their intake of dietary fat, both for weight control and disease prevention. Studies show that a low-fat diet reduces the risk for a variety of cancers, including malignancies of the colon and prostate.

The saturated fat from animal sources, such as butter and red meat, does appear to elevate cancer risk. But the monounsaturated fats in many nuts, as well as in olive and canola oils, and the omega-3 fatty acids in such cold-water fish as salmon and tuna appear to have anticancer effects. They inhibit the body's production of certain inflammatory *prostaglandins*, natural chemicals that can damage cells and initiate changes that lead to cancer.

A study of more than 6,000 Swedish male twins, recently published in the medical journal *The Lancet*, found that men who did not eat fish were two to three times more likely to get prostate cancer than those who ate fish several times a week.

Women who consume large amounts of olive oil may reduce their risk of developing ovarian cancer by 30%. There's also evidence that olive oil, as well as canola oil, lowers breast cancer risk.

SELF-DEFENSE: Limit all dietary fat to 30% or less of total daily calories...use olive or canola oil to replace butter or vegetable oils (which contain less-healthful polyunsaturated fat)...and substitute several weekly servings of fish for red meat or other foods high in saturated fat.

5. Drinking too much alcohol. Although it's true that death rates from cardiovascular disease are lower among men and women who drink moderately than among nondrinkers, the benefits are lost with excessive drinking.

In fact, the death rates from cancers of the mouth, esophagus, larynx and liver in men and women who consume at least four drinks daily are three to seven times higher than among nondrinkers. Women who drink more than one drink a day are at increased risk for breast cancer.

SELF-DEFENSE: Men should consume no more than two drinks daily—women, no more than one. If you have a family history or another risk factor for breast cancer, it's probably best to forgo a daily drink.

6. Getting "safe" tans. Most Americans know that excessive sun exposure increases the risk for skin cancer, but some still believe that tanning beds are a safe alternative. Not true.

People who use tanning beds are 2.5 times more likely to develop *squamous cell carcinoma* (in the main structural cells of the epidermis) and 1.5 times more likely to get *basal cell carcinoma* (in the cells at the lowest layer of the epidermis) than those who don't use them. Some tanning salon sessions expose the body to the same amount of harmful ultraviolet A (UV-A) radiation as an entire day at the beach.

SELF-DEFENSE: If you still want a tan, try sunless tanners, such as those made by Neutrogena or Coppertone, sold in most drugstores.

■

COLON CANCER RISK 50% HIGHER FOR RED MEAT EATERS

Sources: **Michael J. Thun, MD,** head, epidemiological research, American Cancer Society...**Steven H. Zeisel, MD, PhD,** professor of nutrition, American Institute of Cancer Research, and chairman, department of nutrition, both at the University of North Carolina, Chapel Hill...*Journal of the American Medical Association.*

Years of eating a lot of red meat and processed meats, such as salami and pastrami, can increase the risk of colon cancer, researchers report.

THE STUDY...

The 20-year study of more than 148,000 adults between the ages of 50 and 74 defined high consumption of red meat as at least three ounces every day for men, and two ounces daily for women.

High consumption of processed meat was defined as five or six days per week for men, and two or three days per week for women.

The research showed that the risk for colon cancer was 50% greater for the people who had a high consumption of red and processed meat compared with those who ate it no more than three times a week.

Long-term consumption of poultry and fish was associated with a lower risk of colon cancer.

This is not a groundbreaking finding, according to Michael J. Thun, MD, head of epidemiological research at the American Cancer Society (ACS). "There have been 20 such studies looking at the relationship between consumption of red or processed meat and colorectal cancer, and most have shown a greater risk in people with higher consumption," he noted. "But this is the largest study that I'm aware of so far, and it adds substantially to the available evidence."

IMPLICATIONS FOR ATKINS DIETERS...

Also, Dr. Thun said the results of this study should be especially interesting to people who are following the Atkins diet. "The Atkins diet became popular recently, so no one knows the health effects long-term," he said. "But the accumulating evidence that a diet high in red meat or processed meat increases the risk of colon cancer indicates that it would certainly be undesirable to remain on the Atkins diet long-term."

Dr. Thun added, "I haven't eaten red meat for quite a while."

"Moderating red meat intake makes sense in terms of reducing the risk of colon cancer," said Steven H. Zeisel, MD, professor of nutrition at the American Institute of Cancer Research at the University of North Carolina, Chapel Hill.

But because the study findings could be supported by a controlled trial that would follow up people assigned to different diets for years, he isn't ready to forego red meat altogether.

"I don't think that anybody says that eating red meat now and then would increase the risk of cancer. There's no need to become a vegan or make drastic changes in [your] diet. I would be moderating my intake a little more than I would have moderated [it] before," Dr. Zeisel said.

OTHER RISK FACTORS PLAY LARGER ROLE...

Although Dr. Thun believes that "High meat consumption is associated with, at most, a 50% increased risk for cancer of the lower colon," he added that "obesity doubles the risk for all colorectal cancer, as does lack of physical activity."

To reduce colon cancer risk, the ACS recommends people maintain a healthy body weight, get regular physical activity and have regular screenings, including an annual *fecal occult blood test* (FOBT), a colonoscopy every 10 years and a flexible sigmoidoscopy every five years for people older than age 50.

■

DEADLY SKIN CANCER IS ON THE RISE

Source: **Perry Robins, MD,** professor of dermatology at New York University Medical Center, New York City, and founder and president of the Skin Cancer Foundation. *www.skincancer.org.* He is author of *Sun Sense: A Complete Guide to the Prevention, Early Detection and Treatment of Skin Cancer* (Skin Cancer Foundation) and *Understanding Melanoma* (available at many libraries).

Melanoma is the deadliest type of skin cancer. The incidence of melanoma is increasing so fast that it has been called one of the nation's most serious epidemics.

Since 1986, the diagnosis rates of melanoma have more than doubled. This is partly due to an increased awareness of skin cancer. More people are being tested, so more cases are detected. But the real numbers also are rising. The population is aging, and half of adults diagnosed are in their 50s.

Melanoma is more likely than other cancers to spread (metastasize) to other parts of the body. About 12% of patients with melanoma die from the cancer.

IMPORTANT: No one needs to die from skin cancer. With regular screenings, melanoma can be detected and removed before it has a chance to spread.

KNOW THE SIGNS...

Telltale signs of melanoma and other skin cancers...

• *Asymmetrical shape.* Normal moles have a uniform appearance. Moles with irregular shapes are more likely to be cancerous.

• *Border that is irregular.* The edges of the mole might be notched or scalloped.

• *Color changes.* Moles should have a uniform color. If a mole has different colors, it could be melanoma.

• *Diameter.* A mole larger than about one-quarter of an inch (six millimeters) across should be checked.

The Skin Cancer Foundation recommends annual skin exams for people age 40 and over. An exam every three years is enough for younger people. The doctor should examine every inch of skin and note or diagram suspicious moles or skin changes for future evaluation and/or treatment.

CAUSES...

Melanoma occurs in cells (melanocytes) that produce *melanin*, the "tanning" skin pigment. When you spend time in the sun, these cells produce more melanin as a protective mechanism against sun damage. However, excessive sun exposure (along with other, still unknown factors) can damage the DNA in melanocytes and result in cancer.

The sun produces three types of UV radiation. Both UV-A and UV-B rays have been linked to melanocyte damage and melanoma. The third type of radiation, UV-C, is absorbed in the atmosphere and doesn't reach the ground.

Melanomas usually form on parts of the body that aren't regularly exposed to sun. Low levels of melanin in these areas make cells more sensitive to damage. Men tend to develop melanomas on the back. Women are more likely to get them on the legs. Less often, melanomas may occur under a finger- or toenail, in the eye or in mucous membranes that line the nose, mouth, esophagus, anus, urinary tract and vagina.

Heredity also plays a role in melanoma risk. About one out of every 10 patients diagnosed has a family member who has had the disease.

PREVENTION...

Most melanomas can be prevented with simple precautions...

• *Apply sunscreen before going outdoors year-round.* Use it on all exposed skin, including the face, ears, backs of the hands, etc. Apply it a half-hour before going outdoors so that it penetrates the skin and provides maximal protection. Use a product that filters out both UV-A and UV-B rays.

Certain sunscreens may cause a reaction in some people.

SELF-TEST: Apply a small amount to the inside of your arm at night. In the morning, check for a rash, itching or other signs of sensitivity. If there are no changes, the sunscreen should be safe for you.

• *Use a product with an SPF (sun-protection factor) of 30.* Don't pay extra for products with higher SPF numbers—they provide little or no additional protection. Apply a thin layer of sunscreen every two or three hours. Apply it more often if you're swimming or perspiring heavily.

• *Wear protective clothing.* Sunscreens don't completely block UV radiation. Wear a cap or broad-brimmed hat...tightly woven clothing...and sunglasses that block both UV-A and UV-B rays.

• *Stay away from tanning beds.* Some tanning salons advertise that they are safe, but that is not true.

• *Perform monthly self-exams.* Stand in front of a full-length mirror and examine your skin. Use a hand mirror to check hard-to-see areas. Check the soles of your feet and the spaces between your toes, as well as the scalp, groin, etc. New growths...moles that have changed...and sores that don't heal should be checked by a doctor.

■

SPOTS, TAGS, BUMPS: ARE THEY SKIN CANCER?

Source: **Barney J. Kenet, MD,** dermatologist at New York-Presbyterian Hospital Weill Cornell Medical Center in New York City, author of *Saving Your Skin* (Avalon) and cofounder of the American Melanoma Foundation.

As we grow older, various lumps, bumps and spots (skin tags, wart-like growths, brown or black raised spots) come to mar the flawless skin of our youth. Dermatologists sometimes refer to these as the "barnacles of aging." The million-dollar question that everybody asks is—when is a bump just a bump... and when is it a sign of skin cancer?

THREE TYPES OF SKIN CANCER...

Skin cancer is the most common type of cancer in the US, with more than one million new cases diagnosed each year, according to Barney J. Kenet, MD, a New York City dermatologist who specializes in skin cancer. **OF THE NEW CASES EACH YEAR...**

• *80% are basal cell carcinoma.*
• *16% are squamous cell carcinoma.*
• *4% are melanoma.*

Basal cell and squamous cell carcinomas have a cure rate of more than 95%. However, melanoma is a different story. This deadly cancer can spread quickly to organs, such as the liver and lungs, and it accounts for more than three out of four deaths from all skin cancers.

Because even melanoma can be completely cured with early diagnosis and treatment, it's essential to learn the warning signs of skin cancer.

BASAL CELL CARCINOMA...

This most common form of skin cancer first appears as small and occasionally discolored, fleshy nodules or bumps on frequently sun-exposed areas of the body, such as the hands, head or neck. If the lesions occur on the trunk, they are generally flat instead of raised. Slow-growing basal cell carcinomas may take as long as months or even years to reach a diameter of half an inch. Yet this does not mean you should ignore them. Left untreated, they may bleed and crust over again and again, and after years, a neglected lesion can eventually penetrate the bone beneath.

SQUAMOUS CELL CARCINOMA...

The second most common skin cancer may first appear as a pink, tan or brown bump or patch on a sun-exposed area of the skin, or it can develop out of an actinic keratosis (a precancerous condition of rough red or brown scaly patches). Squamous cell tumors are also relatively slow to spread—however, they do grow more quickly than basal cell carcinomas.

This cancer is sometimes difficult to detect in its early stages. At first, squamous cell carcinomas are firm to the touch. As they begin to grow, the tumors form a central crust, which becomes ulcerated and results in the surrounding skin becoming red and inflamed.

Both basal cell and squamous cell cancers most often occur in fair-skinned people who do not tan easily.

MELANOMA...

Melanoma is more common in fair-skinned people. However, it shows up more frequently than basal and squamous cell carcinomas in people of color. This virulent disease is on the rise, affecting a greater number of people every year. Those who have a large number of freckles and moles—especially unusual-looking moles that have uneven textures, margins or coloration that change suddenly in sensitivity, appearance or size—are at the highest risk. Unlike basal and squamous cell cancers, melanoma most commonly occurs on parts of the body that are less frequently exposed to the sun, including the back, trunk, arms and legs.

The American Academy of Dermatology teaches the basics about melanoma. SEE A DERMATOLOGIST IMMEDIATELY IF YOU NOTICE ANY OF THE FOLLOWING CHANGES IN A MOLE OR PIG-MENTED AREA...

• *Asymmetry,* when one half of the mole does not match the other side.

• *Border irregularity,* when edges of the mole are either ragged or notched.

• *Color varied from one area to another* in shades of brown, tan or black, or sometimes red, blue or white.

• *Diameter of greater than 6 millimeters* (the size of the top of a pencil eraser).

SIGNS AND SYMPTOMS OF SKIN CANCER...

Skin cancers do not all look the same. Some are raised, others are flat...some bumps look pale, others are colored.

Warning signs include...

• *A new growth on the skin that does not heal.*

• *Changes in the size or color of a mole* or other pigmented spot.

• *Scaliness, oozing, bleeding or change in the appearance of a bump or nodule.*

• *Tenderness, itchiness or pain* in a skin growth.

VIGILANCE PAYS...

Now that you know what to look for, conduct a thorough skin self-exam once a month. Using a full-length as well as a hand-held mirror, search for any new blemishes or alterations in existing growths. If you detect something suspicious, see your doctor. Remember to look in places that are not usually exposed to the sun, such as in between toes and the soles of feet.

If you're age 40 or older, also visit a dermatologist once a year for a full skin exam, in which you will be checked from head to toe.

BASIC RULE: Early detection and treatment are the secrets to a complete cure.

■

HEPATITIS C RAISES RISK OF NON-HODGKIN'S LYMPHOMA

Source: American Association for Cancer Research news release.

People who are infected with the hepatitis C virus (HCV) are six times more likely to develop non-Hodgkin's lymphoma (NHL) than people who are not infected with the virus, according to a Canadian study.

Researchers examined the HCV status of 550 people who had NHL and 205 healthy control subjects. "People who have been exposed to the virus comprise a high-risk group for developing non-Hodgkin's lymphoma," said John Spinelli, a cancer researcher at the British Columbia Cancer Agency in Vancouver.

Previous studies in Canada and the United States did not find an association between HCV and NHL.

Approximately 3.8 million people in the United States are infected with HCV. In 2003, approximately 23,000 Americans died from the virus. While blood transfusion used to be the most common way people became infected, it is most often transmitted now among drug users who share needles.

The National Center for Infectious Diseases has more information about hepatitis C on its Web site, *www.cdc.gov/ncidod/diseases/hepatitis.*

NON-HODGKIN'S LYMPHOMA SYMPTOMS

Source: The Lancet news release.

The symptom that is most common in non-Hodgkin's lymphoma is a painless swelling of the lymph nodes in the neck, underarm or groin, according the National Cancer Institute. OTHER SYMPTOMS MAY INCLUDE THE FOLLOWING...

- *Unexplained fever.*
- *Night sweats.*
- *Constant fatigue.*

- *Unexplained weight loss.*
- *Itchy skin.*
- *Reddened patches on the skin.*

These symptoms are not sure signs of non-Hodgkin's lymphoma, and could be caused by other, less serious conditions, such as the flu or other infections.

If you experience any of these symptoms, it is important to see a doctor so that any illness can be diagnosed and treated as early as possible. Don't wait to feel pain—early non-Hodgkin's lymphoma may not cause pain.

You can learn more about non-Hodgkin's lymphoma from the National Institutes of Health's Medline Plus at *www.nlm. nih.gov/medlineplus/ency/article/000581.htm.*

■

WORRIED ABOUT SKIN CANCER? CHECK YOUR FEET AND ANKLES FIRST

Sources: Foot and Ankle Surgery...American College of Foot & Ankle Surgery news release.

Melanoma, the deadliest form of skin cancer, is always a concern. But when the disease strikes the feet and ankles, it's particularly lethal.

A study by Rhode Island podiatric foot and ankle surgeon Susan M. Walsh, MD, found that the overall five-year survival rate for people who had primary melanoma of the foot or ankle was 52%, compared with 84% for those people who had melanoma on the thigh or calf.

"The results of this study should serve as a strong reminder for physicians and patients to be vigilant in checking the feet carefully for evidence of skin cancer," Walsh said.

"A malignant melanoma on the foot, especially if it isn't painful and if it's on the bottom of the foot, won't be as readily noticed as a lesion on the face or arm. Foot melanomas, therefore, are more advanced and more dangerous," Walsh said.

RISK FACTORS AND HOW TO PROTECT YOURSELF...

Melanomas can be found anywhere on the foot—even under a toenail. Risk factors for foot and ankle melanomas are similar to other skin cancers, and include excessive sun exposure, family history of skin cancer, numerous moles on the body and having fair skin, blue eyes or red hair.

Doctors should be highly suspicious when a patient has a pigmented or unusual lesion on the foot, Dr. Walsh advised. Anyone with moles on their feet should have the moles removed and biopsied if they change color or shape.

According to the National Cancer Institute, more than 53,000 Americans are diagnosed with melanoma each year, accounting for only 4% of the total number of skin cancers, but causing the vast majority of skin cancer deaths.

■

TIPS FOR SUN PROTECTION

*Sources: Cancer...*John Wiley & Sons, Inc., news release.

The leading risk factor for skin cancer is exposure to sunlight. Sunlight can sometimes cause damage to the DNA that is found in skin cells.

The Skin Cancer Foundation (*www.skincancer.org*) offers the following seven tips for sun safety...

1. *Don't sunbathe.* A tan might seem glamorous, but it's not worth the risk.

2. *Avoid unnecessary exposure to the sun,* especially between the hours of 10 am and 4 pm, the peak period of time for harmful ultraviolet (UV) radiation.

3. *Use sunscreens rated SPF 15 or higher.* Apply them liberally and frequently.

4. *Wear clothing that is protective,* such as long pants, long-sleeved shirts, broad-brimmed hats and UV-protective sunglasses.

5. *Avoid artificial tanning devices.*

6. *Teach your children good sun-protection habits at an early age.* The skin damage that leads to skin cancers in adults often starts in early childhood.

7. *Examine your skin thoroughly from head-to-toe* at least once every three months.

In addition to exposure to the sun, scientists have identified several other risk factors for nonmelanoma skin tumors. These include exposure to certain types of chemicals, such as arsenic, industrial tar, coal and paraffin, as well as exposure to radiation.

People with severe bone infections and inflammatory diseases, smokers and those people who have weakened immune systems—transplant patients, for example—also are at greater risk of the tumors.

■

DIABETES IS BECOMING AN EPIDEMIC

Source: **Anne Peters, MD,** professor of clinical medicine, Keck School of Medicine of the University of Southern California in Los Angeles, and director of the USC clinical diabetes program. She is author of *Conquering Diabetes—A Cutting-Edge, Comprehensive Program for Prevention and Treatment.* Hudson Street.

The US is in the midst of a diabetes epidemic. Twenty million Americans currently have type 2 (often referred to as adult-onset) diabetes, putting them at risk for such serious complications as blindness, kidney failure, heart disease, nerve damage and circulatory failure leading to amputation.

Another 41 million have prediabetes, which can turn into full-blown diabetes. The problem is that people with high blood sugar levels often don't feel any different—which is why one out of three Americans with diabetes don't even know they have the disease.

MAIN REASON FOR THIS EPIDEMIC: More Americans are overweight and physically inactive—both of which make the body less responsive to insulin, the chemical that transports sugar from the bloodstream into the body's various cells. This condition, known as insulin resistance, forces the body to produce more and more insulin in an effort to keep blood sugar within normal limits. Among those with genetic vulnerability (including many people who aren't overweight), this eventually causes the insulin-producing cells of the pancreas to "burn out," leaving the body unable to produce enough insulin to control blood sugar.

THE RESULT: Soaring blood sugar levels.

GOOD NEWS: Complications can be avoided by catching insulin resistance early and then taking basic steps to bring blood sugar levels within normal limits.

GET A FASTING BLOOD SUGAR TEST...

The best way to learn whether you have insulin resistance is a fasting blood sugar test—a simple blood draw, taken 10 to 12 hours after you've last eaten. It should be included in your annual physical. If you haven't had a fasting blood sugar test within the past year, call your primary care physician and schedule one—*especially* if you have a family history of diabetes.

A fasting blood sugar level of 126 milligrams per deciliter (mg/dl) or higher indicates diabetes, while a result between 100 and 125 mg/dl indicates prediabetes.

I always recommend a second test to confirm a high reading. If your test result is below 100, your blood sugar is within normal range, but you still may have early-stage insulin resistance—particularly if you are overweight or have close relatives with diabetes. If you and your doctor suspect this may be the case, you should follow the steps outlined below.

TEST FOR CARDIOVASCULAR RISK FACTORS...

Since insulin resistance is associated with significantly increased risk of heart disease, it's important that your doctor order a cholesterol (lipid) panel and check your blood pressure and body mass index (BMI). Body mass index is a measurement indicating how your weight/height ratio stacks up against the general population.

Triglyceride (a type of blood lipid) levels above 150 mg/dl and HDL (good) cholesterol levels below 50 (for women) or 40 (men), blood pressure of more than 115/75 and a BMI over 25 are all signs that you may be at risk for both heart disease and prediabetes/diabetes.

DEVELOP A TREATMENT PLAN WITH YOUR DOCTOR...

Some doctors still believe that there's nothing to worry about as long as your blood sugar is less than 126. However, if one of my patients has a fasting blood sugar above 100 (or less than 100, but with other risk factors for insulin resistance or a family history of diabetes), I generally treat that patient as if he/she already has diabetes.

REASON: Damage from insulin resistance starts long before blood sugar reaches "diabetic" levels.

This is why I urge everybody to ask their doctors for copies of their blood test results, rather than take a doctor's word that everything is OK. If your blood sugar is above 100, you need to discuss setting up a treatment plan with your doctor, or find another doctor if yours isn't responsive. **THIS PLAN SHOULD INCLUDE FIVE ELEMENTS...**

- *Lose weight and exercise.*
- *Reduce cardiac risk associated with diabetes.* This includes taking a baby aspirin daily to reduce risk of heart attack and stroke, and, if your test results warrant, a statin drug (Lipitor, Zocor, Crestor) to lower high cholesterol, fibric acid derivatives (Lopid, Tricor) to lower triglycerides and ACE inhibitors (Lotensin, Vasotec, Zestril, Altace) or angiotensin receptor blockers (Avapro, Cozaar, Hyzaar, Diovan) to treat high blood pressure.
- *Test blood sugar regularly.* If your fasting blood sugar test is above 100, I recommend getting another fasting blood sugar test every three months.

If your blood sugar test is above 125, you'll need to test more often. My diabetic patients do home blood tests every day, including first thing in the morning and two hours after each meal, and also get an A1C blood test every three months. This test shows what your average blood sugar level was for the previous several months. The goal is to keep your A1C below 7, and preferably between 4 and 6.

- *Consider diabetes medication.* If your blood sugar levels continue to be high despite weight loss and exercise, you and your doctor might consider *glitazone* medication—either *pioglitazone* (Actos) or *rosiglitazone* (Avandia)—to increase your body's sensitivity to insulin.

Your doctor may also prescribe *metformin* (which reduces the liver's glucose production and can be used with glitazones) and/or alpha-glucosidase inhibitors, such as *acarbose* (Precose) or *miglitol* (Glyset), which decrease the amount of carbohydrates absorbed by the intestines. (Unfortunately, they also tend to produce large amounts of intestinal gas.) Also, the new injected drug *exenatide* (Byetta) can help lower blood sugar level and weight at the same time.

If all else fails, your doctor can prescribe daily insulin doses to supplement your body's natural insulin production.

• *Test for complications of insulin resistance.* Since cell damage from diabetes begins early, I also recommend regular tests for complications, even if your blood sugar is only slightly elevated.

REASON: Diabetes-related complications may be treatable early on, but once damage becomes serious, treatment becomes difficult or impossible.

TESTS INCLUDE: An annual dilated eye exam by an ophthalmologist...a yearly urine test for microalbuminuria (an early sign of kidney damage)...yearly cholesterol and triglyceride tests...a check for normal foot sensation at every doctor's visit, and if numbness is detected, twice daily home foot exams for cuts or sores that you can't feel.

THE KEY TO DIABETES PREVENTION...

Losing weight is the single most effective way to prevent developing diabetes.

REASON: Putting on even as little as 10 pounds—especially around your middle—automatically increases insulin resistance. Losing just 15 pounds reduces your risk of developing diabetes by more than half.

A SIMPLE, PROVEN WAY TO LOSE WEIGHT: Eat smaller portions. Use small (10-inch) plates at home—and therefore serve smaller portions—since studies show that people tend to finish whatever is on their plates. Also, avoid fruit juices and soft drinks as well as "white" foods (white bread, baked potatoes and French fries, pasta, white rice), all of which cause sharp rises in blood sugar. Finally, make sure that every meal contains a mix of high-fiber fruits and vegetables and high-quality protein (fish or lean meat).

ANOTHER KEY: Do an hour of exercise at least five times a week. A good program for most people is 45 minutes of aerobic exercise—such as walking, biking or swimming—and 15 minutes of light weight lifting.

REASON: Regular exercise encourages weight loss and increases your body's sensitivity to insulin. This effect only lasts a short time, however, which is why it's important to exercise often.

For many, these steps will be enough to prevent diabetes. If your body's ability to respond to insulin is 75% of normal and you can lower your insulin resistance by 25% through diet and exercise—a typical response—then your blood-sugar regulation will be brought back in balance.

■

WARNING: SOME DIABETES DRUGS MAY CAUSE HEART PROBLEMS

Sources: **Abhimanyu Garg, MD,** professor, internal medicine, University of Texas Southwestern Medical Center, Dallas...*Mayo Clinic Proceedings.*

Type 2 diabetics with mild heart disease or kidney problems could increase their risk of developing congestive heart failure by taking certain diabetes medications, according to research.

The study examined six cases of congestive heart failure in people taking *pioglitazone* (Actos) or *rosiglitazone* (Avandia) to help control their diabetes.

"We could not identify any other reason for the deterioration of their status," said the lead author of the study, Abhimanyu Garg, MD, a professor of internal medicine at the University of Texas Southwestern Medical Center located in Dallas.

Because these medications are known to cause fluid accumulation, doctors discontinued them and gave the patients diuretics to help flush excess fluid from the body. All responded to this treatment.

The current study, he said, confirmed what is already known about these medications.

THE CASES...

The researchers studied the records of six men, between the ages of 66 and 78 years, with type 2 diabetes who had gone to the emergency room at Dallas Veterans Affairs Medical Center.

All six complained of shortness of breath, swelling of their feet and weight gain, which are symptoms of congestive heart failure and pulmonary edema (fluid buildup in the lungs).

Congestive heart failure occurs when the heart can no longer pump enough blood to maintain adequate circulation. Because the heart doesn't pump properly, fluid often builds up in the lungs.

These drugs are not recommended for people with more advanced heart disease—the type that causes physical limitations.

Four of the six people in this study had chronic renal insufficiency, which means that their kidneys weren't functioning normally. Only two of the participants had any previous signs of heart disease. Four of the six had high blood pressure.

All of the study subjects had been taking the diabetes medications for between one month and 16 months. Three of the participants developed symptoms within one to three months after the dose of their diabetes drug had been increased.

The authors conclude that anyone with a history of congestive heart failure or chronic kidney disease should avoid taking these medications, and they suggest that further study be done on them.

"If somebody is taking these medications and they develop severe swelling or severe weight gain, they are not tolerating the medication," said Dr. Garg, who recommends seeing a doctor immediately if you or someone you know is experiencing any of these symptoms.

■

SUDDEN CARDIAC DEATH MAY START WITH STRESS

Source: University College London news release.

Disrupted signals from the brain to the heart may be responsible for the type of sudden cardiac death that is caused by emotional stress, according to a University College London study.

The study found that some people have problems with the system that coordinates signals sent from the brain stem to different parts of the heart to control heart rhythm. These people may have a greater risk of potentially fatal heart rhythms when they're performing stressful mental tasks or during emotional events.

Researchers came to this conclusion after monitoring people with heart disease while they performed stressful mental tasks. Stress-induced changes in heart electrical currents were accompanied by uneven activity within the brain stem, they found.

"Some people are at risk of sudden cardiac death from stress, mainly people who already have heart disease. In these cases, the combination of heart and brain irregularities means heart failure could occur during a stressful or emotional event like a family gathering or even a boisterous New Year's party," according to researcher Dr. Peter Taggart of the University's Centre for Cardiology.

"Efforts to prevent the development of potentially dangerous heart rhythms in response to stress have focused on drugs which act directly on the heart, but results have so far been rather disappointing," he added. "Our research focuses on what is happening...in the brain, when stress causes these heart rhythm problems. The results so far are very encouraging."

The Heart Rhythm Society has more information about sudden cardiac death at *www.hrspatients.org/patients*.

DON'T IGNORE CHEST PAIN—EVER!...

Many people get a little chest pain once in a while. Others get a lot of chest pain too often.

Pain in the chest caused by insufficient blood and oxygen to the heart is called *angina pectoris*. Because angina could indicate that a heart attack is imminent, doctors consider all serious chest pain to be heart-related until proven otherwise.

Fortunately, the majority of chest pain stems from something other than arterial blockages severe enough to cause angina pectoris and a heart attack, according to the Centers for Disease Control and Prevention (CDC).

Other causes of chest pain can include...

• *A pinched nerve in the neck.*

• *Viral inflammation* of ribs and cartilage.

• *Diseases of the ribs,* the lungs (pneumonia, other infections, cancer, etc.) and the lungs' covering (pleurisy).

- *Diseases of the breathing pipe.*

- *Diseases of the esophagus* (food pipe).

- *Chest muscle spasm.*

- *Muscle injury.*

- *Arthritis of the spine* or almost any joint in the chest area.

- *Diseases of the diaphragm* (the muscular "tent" that separates the chest cavity from the abdominal cavity, dividing them into two airtight compartments).

If you experience chest pain, don't take chances—check with your physician.

■

HEART DISEASE, THE #1 KILLER OF WOMEN

Source: **Harvey S. Hecht, MD, FACC,** director, preventive cardiology, Continuum Heart Institute of Beth Israel Medical Center, New York City, and past president of the Society for Atherosclerosis Imaging.

With all the fund-raising and public relations efforts surrounding breast cancer, women often overlook their number-one killer—heart disease. The reality is that one-third of all women develop cardiovascular problems by age 45. And each year, more women die from heart disease than from the next seven causes of death combined. We naively think of cardiac issues as a male problem. Not even close.

To learn more about the special challenges women face with heart disease and what to do about them, Harvey S. Hecht, MD, FACC, director of preventive cardiology at the Continuum Heart Institute of Beth Israel Medical Center, located in New York City, and past president of the Society for Atherosclerosis Imaging, provided the following information.

VAGUE SYMPTOMS CAN BE MISLEADING...

A major concern is that women experience much more subtle heart attack symptoms than do men, explained Dr. Hecht. In place of or in addition to chest discomfort, women may have shortness of breath, fatigue, back discomfort, nausea and dizziness. These complaints are often underestimated by both women and their doctors or are mistaken for signs of other disorders.

Dr. Hecht warned that this is a life-threatening error, as timing is everything when it comes to heart attack intervention. The sooner the treatment, the better your chances of survival. The hope is that women will team up with their doctors to prevent heart disease, and with increased awareness, they will also be better equipped to recognize dangerous warning signs.

NEW HEART-HEALTHY GUIDELINES...

Finally dispensing with the one-size-fits-all perspective, the American Heart Association (AHA) issued new guidelines to aggressively reduce the risk for heart disease and stroke in women. The guidelines urge women to get regular heart checkups, during which blood pressure and cholesterol levels are evaluated, just as they get regular breast exams...and to treat risk factors, such as high blood cholesterol and high blood pressure, at lower thresholds than in the past.

The new guidelines base the aggressiveness of treatment on whether a woman is at a low, intermediate or high degree of risk for heart attack within the next 10 years, according to a standardized scoring method developed by the Framingham Heart Study in Massachusetts.

Risk is based on such factors as age, blood pressure, cholesterol levels and smoking status. Low risk means that a woman has a less than 10% chance of suffering a heart attack within the next 10 years...intermediate risk is a 10% to 20% chance... and high risk means that a woman is at a greater than 20% risk of suffering a heart attack within the next 10 years.

The AHA's recommendations include...

• *All women should be assessed for their heart disease risk* beginning as early as age 20. They should get regular heart checkups along with their annual physical exam from a physician.

• *If blood pressure measures 140/90 or higher,* women should take antihypertensive (blood-pressure-lowering) medication.

• *Because of the risk of bleeding,* strokes and stomach problems, only women at high risk should take aspirin daily.

• *Women should not take hormone replacement therapy (HRT) to prevent heart disease.* Recent studies have indicated that

HRT may actually have harmful consequences to women's cardiovascular health, noted Dr. Hecht.

• *Since they have shown no individual heart-healthy benefits in several large clinical trials,* the guidelines are not in favor of beta-carotene or vitamin E supplements.

• *All women should follow a healthy diet,* get regular exercise and refrain from smoking.

EARLY SCREENING IS OPTIMAL...

Dr. Hecht is also a strong believer in early screening and treatment. He is a leader in the development of electron beam tomography (EBT), a non-invasive screening tool that does not use needles or dyes, and is 98% accurate in detecting coronary artery disease in its earliest stages. It is now available in most major cities. The scan works by detecting the presence of coronary calcium, an indicator of plaque. When plaque composed of fatty cholesterol and calcium deposits accumulates on the walls of arteries, blood vessels narrow and can rupture, causing a heart attack.

Dr. Hecht recommends EBT for all women over the age of 55... women age 45 and over with any risk factors...and women under age 45 with a striking family history of premature heart disease (such as a parent, brother or sister who had a heart attack).

Early screening also makes early intervention possible, and Dr. Hecht is a strong advocate of "interventional lipidology," a practice that combines early detection of coronary atherosclerosis by EBT with aggressive drug treatment of cholesterol disorders.

PREVENTION AND INTERVENTION: THE EARLIER, THE BETTER...

To prevent heart disease, Dr. Hecht recommends adhering to a heart-healthy diet, exercise, weight control and no smoking. If screening indicates that a woman is at high risk for a heart attack, he strongly advises taking more aggressive measures, such as cholesterol control. If symptoms of a heart attack occur, remember that every second counts—call 911 and get immediate assistance.

WARNING SIGNS OF HEART ATTACK ARE DIFFERENT FOR WOMEN

Source: **Jean McSweeney, PhD, RN,** professor, University of Arkansas for Medical Sciences, Little Rock, and lead researcher of a survey of 515 female heart attack survivors, published in *Circulation.*

Women may experience heart attack warning symptoms more than a month before they have an attack. The most common symptom is overwhelming fatigue, reported by 71% of women.

Other reported symptoms are sleep disturbance (48%), shortness of breath (42%), indigestion (39%) and anxiety (35%). Only 30% experience chest discomfort.

SELF-DEFENSE: If you are experiencing these or any suspicious symptoms, contact your doctor.

TROUBLE BREATHING?

Source: **Daniel S. Berman, MD,** director of cardiac imaging/nuclear cardiology, Cedars-Sinai Heart Center, Los Angeles, and leader of a study of 17,991 patients, published in *New England Journal of Medicine.*

According to research, shortness of breath may indicate heart disease—especially if it is a new symptom in someone age 50 or older.

NEW STUDY: People with unexplained breathing problems have more than twice the risk of dying from cardiac causes as people who report chest pain.

REASON: Patients who experience chest pain are more likely to be treated.

SELF-DEFENSE: If you experience shortness of breath, contact your doctor.

ED MAY MEAN HEART PROBLEMS

Source: **Alan J. Bank, MD,** director of research, St. Paul Heart Clinic, St. Paul, MN.

Erectile dysfunction (ED) affects some 30 million men in this country. In years past, most people—including many doctors—assumed that the cause of ED was almost always psychological or a side effect of medication.

We now know, though, that in the vast majority of cases, the cause of ED is vascular—an inability of the penile vessels to engorge with blood. It is also well established that ED and cardiovascular disease share risk factors—smoking, high blood pressure, uncontrolled cholesterol levels, obesity and type 2 diabetes. Doctors have associated ED with late-stage cardiovascular disease. Research shows that more than half of the men who come to the hospital with a heart attack or stroke report having had ED.

Recent research on ED has come to the intriguing conclusion that ED may actually serve as an early warning symptom for some types of cardiovascular disease.

The study's author, Alan J. Bank, MD, director of research at the St. Paul Heart Clinic in Minnesota, discussed his study and its implications. He explained that the purpose of the study was to evaluate men who suffered from ED but who were otherwise healthy. The 30 study participants were all relatively young (mean age 46) nonsmokers who were reasonably fit, and who had no other cardiovascular disease risk factors or symptoms of disease.

STUDY DETAILS...

The researchers examined the chemical pathway of a substance called *nitric oxide* (NO)—produced by the smooth lining of the arteries (the endothelium)—which causes artery walls to dilate and relax. An abnormality in the NO system is an early stage of artery disease (atherosclerosis) because NO is instrumental in the healthy functioning of all arteries in the body, including those linked to ED.

Researchers first established that the study participants' ED resulted from a malfunction of the NO system in the penile vessels. They then examined the NO chemical pathway in other arteries. They found no problem in the men's aorta, carotid artery leading to the brain and the cardiac arteries, but when they looked at the NO pathway in the brachial artery, a vessel in the upper arm, they found a malfunction. This established that the vascular malfunction was broader than that which caused the ED in these patients.

WHAT IT MEANS...

What this means for some men who have ED, including those who are seemingly healthy and without risk for cardiac disease, is that they should take immediate steps to bolster their cardiac health, according to Dr. Bank. He recommends that they inform their doctors about this observed link and work together to make lifestyle changes, such as nutritional therapy, that enhance cardiac health, and, if necessary, to consider appropriate medication. Reducing stress and enhancing sleep quality are examples of nonpharmaceutical interventions.

Improve your health and your symptoms will be less problematic...and any cardiac-enhancing medication, if needed, will work better and also with fewer side effects.

■

EVEN MILD DEPRESSION MAY INCREASE HEART FAILURE RISK

Sources: **Wei Jiang, MD,** assistant professor of internal medicine and psychiatry, Duke University Medical Center, Durham, NC...American College of Cardiology scientific sessions, Orlando, FL...American Psychosomatic Society annual meeting, Vancouver ...Duke University press release...Duke University Medical Center news release.

A state of depression so mild that most doctors might not notice it significantly increases the long-term risk of death for people who have heart failure, a study has found.

After tracking 1,005 heart failure patients for seven years, researchers found that those who were identified as mildly depressed based on their score on a standard psychiatric test were 44% more likely to die compared with people who scored in the normal range.

Surprisingly, the death rate was higher—51%—for patients whose score indicated somewhat milder depression.

Wei Jiang, MD, an assistant professor of internal medicine and psychiatry at Duke University Medical Center, said that she undertook the study because other trials have linked depression to an increased risk of death from other cardiac conditions, such as heart attacks.

Patients were given the Beck's Depression Inventory (BDI), a test that asks people to rate the veracity of 21 statements, such as "I am disappointed in myself" and "I hate myself."

People who have a BDI score of 10 are considered mildly depressed. The 44% increase in mortality in the study was recorded for people who scored 10 or higher. However, the 51% increase in mortality was found in people who scored only 7 or higher, Jiang noted.

"The majority of patients in our study would not be regarded as having clinical depression," said Dr. Jiang.

It's not known why depression is related to greater risk of death, but some research has linked it to physical effects—such as a decreased ability of the heart to respond to the stresses of everyday life. In addition, depressed people are more likely to miss doctors' appointments and less likely to stick with exercise programs and drug regimens, Dr. Jiang said. Depressed patients may also make unhealthy lifestyle choices, such as smoking and not following a proper diet.

THE LESSON: Doctors should pay close attention to heart patients' psychological outlook, Dr. Jiang recommended.

■

HOW TO PREVENT A STROKE

Source: **Patrick Lyden, MD,** professor of neurosciences and director of the Stroke Center at University of California, San Diego. He is also chief of the Stroke Clinic at the San Diego VA Medical Center.

Stroke is the most *preventable* cause of death and disability in the United States. Yet more than 750,000 Americans suffer strokes each year...about 160,000 of these people die... and approximately 200,000 people live with lasting disability. What are we doing wrong?

You can't change some risk factors, such as family history. If you have a parent or sibling who has suffered a stroke, you are at greater risk yourself.

Your age also plays a role. And although strokes can occur even in young children, overall risk steadily increases as we grow older. That's why more than two-thirds of strokes occur in people over age 65.

Beyond these factors, whether or not we suffer a stroke is largely up to us.

WHAT IS A STROKE?...

A stroke occurs when blood supply to a part of the brain is interrupted. Without oxygen and nutrients, brain cells die within minutes, damaging areas that control movement, speech—and even involuntary activities, such as breathing.

STROKE PREVENTION...

What most affects stroke risk...

• *Smoking.* Everyone knows that smoking increases heart disease risk, but did you know that smoking is actually more likely to cause a *stroke* than a heart attack?

Not only does smoking promote the development of fatty deposits that narrow arteries (atherosclerosis), but the nicotine in tobacco causes blood vessels in the brain to constrict.

RESULT: Smokers have up to four times the stroke risk of nonsmokers.

WHAT YOU CAN DO: Quit smoking. If you've tried but can't kick the habit, consider using nicotine-replacement patches or gum...or the prescription drug *bupropion* (Zyban).

• *Blood pressure.* High blood pressure gradually damages blood vessels and substantially increases the risk for both ischemic strokes (a blood clot stops blood supply to an area of the brain) and hemorrhagic strokes (a broken or leaking blood vessel causes bleeding into or around the brain). The risk is greater because high blood pressure rarely causes symptoms, so the problem goes unrecognized in 30% of sufferers.

WHAT YOU CAN DO: If your blood pressure exceeds 115/75, take steps to reduce it. Weight loss and exercise may be enough, but you also may need to take medication, such as diuretics or beta blockers.

• *Cholesterol.* For stroke prevention, maintain the same cholesterol levels that are recommended to reduce heart disease risk—total cholesterol under 200...LDL "bad" cholesterol under 80...HDL "good" cholesterol above 40.

WHAT YOU CAN DO: Weight loss and exercise help control cholesterol levels. If these strategies are insufficient, cholesterol-lowering medication may be needed.

• *Diabetes.* Maintaining very tight control of blood sugar (glucose) will help to minimize small blood vessel damage that can lead to stroke.

WHAT YOU CAN DO: Work with your doctor to create a treatment plan that keeps your hemoglobin A1C (average blood sugar over time) level at less than seven.

• *Diet.* Stroke risk, like heart disease risk, can be related to what foods you consume.

WHAT YOU CAN DO: Maintain a diet that's low in saturated fats (no more than 30% of total fats per day) and high in fruits and vegetables (five to nine one-half cup servings per day).

Research shows that people who are deficient in potassium are 1.5 to 2.5 times more likely to have a stroke. Aim for the government's recommended potassium intake of 4,700 milligrams (mg) daily. Although bananas are a popular source of potassium (one medium banana contains 457 mg of potassium), cantaloupe can be an even richer source (one cup of cantaloupe balls contains about 547 mg).

If you determine that sodium raises your blood pressure, limit your daily sodium intake to 2.4 grams (g) (slightly more than one teaspoon of salt).

• *Exercise.* Physical activity reduces risk for heart disease, diabetes and hypertension—and may offer stroke protection as well.

WHAT YOU CAN DO: Work with your doctor to create an exercise program based on your history of heart disease, smoking, etc.

• *Daily aspirin.* Aspirin reduces the tendency of platelets to clump, which helps prevent blood clots that can sometimes lead to ischemic stroke.

WHAT YOU CAN DO: If you're over age 55 and have diabetes, high cholesterol or other stroke risk factors, ask your doctor about starting daily low-dose (81-mg) aspirin therapy.

In patients who have never had a stroke or heart attack, and who do not have hypertension, diabetes or elevated cholesterol, the risk of hemorrhage may outweigh the potential benefits of aspirin.

• *Alcohol.* Moderate drinking has been shown to benefit the heart, but it does not curb stroke risk.

WHAT YOU CAN DO: Men should limit alcohol intake to two drinks per day...one drink per day for women. A drink is defined as 1.5 ounces of hard liquor, 4 ounces of wine or 12 ounces of beer. Risk for hemorrhagic stroke jumps substantially if you exceed this amount.

OTHER RISK FACTORS...

Some medical conditions significantly raise your stroke risk...

• *Atrial fibrillation.* About 2.2 million Americans are affected by atrial fibrillation (AF), a heart rhythm disturbance that increases stroke risk five- to sixfold.

AF can cause dizziness, shortness of breath and constriction or other uncomfortable sensations in the chest. Or it may cause no symptoms and be found during a routine examination or when you have an electrocardiogram.

WHAT YOU CAN DO: Taking a blood-thinning drug, such as *warfarin* (Coumadin), can virtually eliminate AF's added stroke risk by preventing the formation of blood clots. Aspirin may be nearly as effective.

• *Transient ischemic attack (TIA).* If you have had one or more of these brief stroke-like episodes, your risk for a full-blown stroke increases dramatically. A TIA can cause dizziness, numbness or paralysis on one side of the body, difficulty speaking, double vision or other stroke symptoms that disappear after minutes or hours.

WHAT YOU CAN DO: After a TIA, ask your doctor about taking antiplatelet medication, such as aspirin, *clopidogrel* (Plavix) or aspirin-*dipyridamole* (Aggrenox).

• *Carotid stenosis.* When fatty deposits accumulate in the carotid artery, which carries blood up through the neck, they can impede brain circulation enough to cause a stroke. Up to half of all ischemic strokes are associated with carotid stenosis.

WHAT YOU CAN DO: If you have had a stroke or TIA, get an ultrasound of your carotid artery. If blockage is 70% or more, ask your doctor about surgery.

■

BEST WAYS TO CUT YOUR STROKE RISK

Source: **Ralph L. Sacco, MS, MD,** professor of neurology and epidemiology, Columbia University Medical Center, New York City, and a national spokesperson for the American Stroke Association. *www.strokeassociation.org.*

Every year, approximately 750,000 Americans experience strokes. Although quick treatment using clot-busting drugs can sharply reduce the damage caused by a stroke, treatments must be given within the early hours of the stroke's occurrence.

Only 1% to 2% of US stroke victims arrive at a hospital in time to get treated with anticlotting medication. So it is even more important that people do their best to prevent strokes. They can do this by lowering or eliminating their stroke risk factors. **HERE ARE THE MAJOR RISK FACTORS THAT CAN (AND CAN'T) BE CHANGED AND HOW TO MANAGE THEM EFFECTIVELY...**

RISK FACTORS YOU CAN'T AVOID...

There's nothing you can do about some risk factors. The more you have, the more vigilant you need to be about those that you can control. **NON-MODIFIABLE FACTORS INCLUDE...**

• *Age.* The risk of stroke goes up steadily with age.

• *Gender.* Since women usually live longer than men, they experience more disability and deaths from stroke.

• *Race and ethnicity.* African-Americans are two times more likely to both have a stroke and die from one than white Americans are. The stroke risk among Hispanic-Americans also appears to be nearly double that of white Americans in the same communities.

• *Genetic background.* If your father, mother or sibling has had a stroke, you may be at elevated risk as well.

RISK FACTORS YOU CAN MANAGE...

Here are the major stroke risk factors that can be managed, and how to handle them...

• *High blood pressure (hypertension) is the biggest risk factor of all.* Clinical studies have shown conclusively that when high blood pressure is lowered, risk of stroke is also reduced.

RISK-REDUCTION STRATEGY: While a low-sodium diet and 30 minutes of daily exercise can help control blood pressure, most people who have hypertension (defined as blood pressure of

140/90 or higher) also require medication, such as beta-blockers, calcium-channel blockers or diuretics, to reach a "normal" blood pressure of 120/80.

People who have moderately elevated blood pressure (121–139/81–89) should seek treatment if they're overweight or have other stroke risk factors.

There's also growing evidence that achieving a blood pressure even lower than 120/80 reduces stroke risk even more.

• *Diabetes.* Having diabetes—defined as a fasting blood sugar level of 126 mg/dL or higher—increases risk of stroke due to increased incidence of small and large blood vessel disease.

RISK-REDUCTION STRATEGY: Work closely with your doctor to manage your blood sugar levels through diet, exercise, regular blood-sugar testing and taking insulin, if necessary. For people with other stroke risk factors, treatment may even be warranted at prediabetic blood sugar levels (more than 110 mg/dL).

• *High LDL ("bad") cholesterol.* While elevated blood cholesterol hasn't been directly linked to increased stroke risk (as it has to coronary artery disease), evidence suggests that people who take statins to lower their LDL cholesterol may also reduce stroke risk.

RISK-REDUCTION STRATEGY: Take statins, maintain a low-fat diet and exercise to boost HDL ("good") cholesterol. For people at low stroke risk, the LDL target is typically 160 mg/dL. With several risk factors present, the target drops to 130. For those at high risk for a stroke, the target might be 100 or even 70.

• *High triglycerides (a blood lipid).* Triglyceride levels of 150 mg/dL or higher have been shown to increase stroke risk in people with preexisting heart disease.

RISK-REDUCTION STRATEGY: Maintain a low-fat diet and take triglyceride-lowering medication, such as statins and fibrates (another group of cholesterol-lowering drugs).

• *Other heart ailments.* Atrial fibrillation, congestive heart failure and valvular heart disease all have been linked to an increased stroke risk.

RISK-REDUCTION STRATEGY: Prompt diagnosis and treatment. Also, possibly, the use of blood thinners such as warfarin.

• *Prior stroke or heart attack.* Someone who has had a stroke is at much greater risk of having another. Heart attack survivors are also at increased risk for stroke.

RISK-REDUCTION STRATEGY: Aspirin and other antiplatelet drugs significantly reduce the risk of experiencing another stroke or heart attack.

• *Cigarette smoking.* Smoking increases stroke risk significantly, in part because smoking damages the walls of the blood vessels, making formation of stroke-causing blood clots more likely.

RISK-REDUCTION STRATEGY: Quit immediately.

• *Heavy alcohol use.* Up to two alcoholic drinks a day for men and one for women may help to *reduce* risk of stroke. Drink more than that, however, and the pendulum begins to swing in the other direction.

For women and men, more than five drinks a day raises stroke risk by increasing the blood's tendency to clot (and contributes to hypertension and heart and liver disease).

RISK-REDUCTION STRATEGY: Men should limit themselves to two drinks per day...women, one drink.

• *Physical inactivity and obesity.* Being overweight, inactive or both increases not only stroke risk, but also your risk for high blood pressure, high cholesterol, heart disease and diabetes.

RISK-REDUCTION STRATEGY: A diet that is restricted in calories. Thirty minutes of aerobic exercise, most or all days of the week.

• *Plaque in the carotid arteries.* Almost 20% of all strokes occur when the carotid arteries are blocked by a blood clot. These arteries are located in the neck and supply blood to the brain. This is more likely to occur in people whose carotid arteries are narrowed by plaque buildup.

RISK-REDUCTION STRATEGY: Diagnostic tests include ultrasound scans, angiograms and magnetic resonance angiograms. Treatments include medication (anticoagulants, antiplatelets, statins or other lipid-lowering drugs) and surgical procedures (*endarterectomy*—surgery to clean out the carotid artery—and angioplasty or stenting).

• *Transient ischemic attacks (TIAs).* TIAs are "warning strokes" or "ministrokes." Treating a TIA promptly by getting urgent medical attention can reduce your risk of a full-blown stroke.

RISK-REDUCTION STRATEGY: Learn the warning signs of a TIA or stroke. Call 911 and get to a hospital immediately.

HIGH BLOOD PRESSURE FACTS...

Approximately 65 million American adults have high blood pressure, according to the National Heart, Lung, and Blood Institute (NHLBI).

Hypertension is often called the "silent killer" because it usually has no symptoms but leads to an increased risk for heart attack, congestive heart failure, stroke and kidney failure.

The NHLBI can tell you more about how to lower your blood pressure at *www.nhlbi.nih.gov/hbp.*

■

STOPPING ASPIRIN CAN TRIPLE STROKE RISK

Sources: **Alexandre Maulaz, MD,** fellow, Stroke Unit, Centre Hospitalier Universitaire de Vaud, Lausanne, Switzerland...**William Buxton, MD,** neurologist, Santa Monica-UCLA Medical Center, Santa Monica, CA, and assistant clinical professor of neurology, David Geffen School of Medicine, UCLA, Los Angeles...American Stroke Association International Stroke Conference, New Orleans.

Stroke survivors who stop taking daily aspirin as recommended by their physicians triple their risk of having another stroke within just one month, researchers say.

Although the exact reasons for this sudden increase in danger are unknown, Swiss investigators speculate that stopping aspirin increases blood platelet activity that is linked to stroke-inducing clots.

THE STUDY...

Researchers in Lausanne, Switzerland, evaluated 309 patients who had experienced a recent stroke or a transient ischemic attack (TIA), also known as a ministroke. All of the patients were placed on long-term 100- or 300-milligram (mg) daily aspirin regimens to help prevent a heart attack or repeated episodes of stroke.

The researchers also evaluated a control group of 309 patients who had had a stroke or TIA more than six months before the study and were already on aspirin therapy due to risk factors, such as high blood pressure or coronary heart disease.

Risk factors in each group were similar, with 69% having high blood pressure, 20% diagnosed with diabetes and 14% smokers. Twice as many individuals (36%) in the recent stroke group had heart disease, compared with the control group (18%). Similar numbers of people in both groups were taking either 100 mg or 300 mg of aspirin daily.

RESULTS...

Among the patients with a recent stroke history, 13 of them had stopped taking daily aspirin in the month preceding their stroke. In contrast, just four patients in the other group had stopped taking aspirin.

This leads the researchers to conclude that those who had had a recent stroke were more than three times as likely to have stopped their aspirin therapy than those who had similar risk factors, but no new stroke or TIA.

While 77% of the ischemic strokes (in which blood flow to the brain is decreased) related to discontinuing aspirin occurred in the first eight days after the aspirin was stopped, the other 23% occurred from day nine through day 30, the researchers report.

THEORIES...

The study findings do not surprise William Buxton, MD, a neurologist on staff at Santa Monica-UCLA Medical Center, and an assistant clinical professor of neurology at the David Geffen School of Medicine at the University of California, Los Angeles. "The study reinforces a lot of our suspicions that going off aspirin or other anti-platelet medications, even for a short time, may put people at risk of stroke," he said.

Study co-researcher Alexandre Maulaz, MD, of the Centre Hospitalier Universitaire de Vaud, Lausanne, speculated that discontinuing aspirin may boost blood platelet numbers and lead to more clotting.

However, he pointed out that both groups in the study had stroke risk factors at the outset. "The possible risk of stroke after stopping aspirin was greater only in patients with many cardiovascular risk factors," he said, "mainly ischemic heart disease. This conclusion cannot be extrapolated for all kinds of persons who take aspirin."

RISKS vs. BENEFITS...

Although most patients who are prescribed stroke prevention therapy are vigilant about following it, Dr. Buxton said, sometimes an upcoming surgery will require patients to discontinue their aspirin therapy. "If you have to go off aspirin therapy before surgery, the doctor must weigh the benefits and risks," he said.

The study points out the importance of following doctor's orders to take aspirin daily and not to change the regimen without permission, Dr. Maulaz said.

■

STROKE SYMPTOMS ARE DIFFERENT FOR MEN AND WOMEN

Sources: **Jaume Roquer, MD, PhD,** physician-researcher, Servei de Neurologia, Hospital del Mar, Barcelona, Spain...**Lewis Morgenstern, MD,** director, stroke center, University of Michigan, Ann Arbor...**Rosabel Young, MD, MS,** clinical assistant professor of neurology, David Geffen School of Medicine, UCLA, Los Angeles.

Some people consider stroke to be a men's health problem. But statistics prove that's not the case.

Strokes kill an estimated 170,000 Americans annually—and about 97,000 of those cases are women, according to the American Heart Association.

It is true, however, that women and men often experience markedly different symptoms. This may make it difficult to diagnose strokes in women, and possibly delay treatment, according to research.

Most stroke patients describe roughly the same general collection of symptoms, including slurred speech, facial paralysis, dizziness and various sensory problems.

THE STUDY...

Jaume Roquer, MD, PhD, a researcher at the Servei de Neurologia at the Hospital del Mar in Barcelona, Spain, and his colleagues evaluated 722 women and 809 men admitted to a hospital for a first stroke between 1995 and 2000. Women were more likely than men to have problems with speech and vision and have difficulties swallowing and chewing. Their hospital stays averaged 15.4 days, compared with 13.4 for men. Women were more disabled after their strokes, too.

However, women are about 60% more likely than men to report other symptoms not generally associated with strokes, such as limb pain, disorientation and fluctuations in consciousness, said Lewis Morgenstern, MD, a stroke specialist at the University of Michigan.

In Roquer's study, the women had higher rates of an irregular heart rhythm known as atrial fibrillation, in which the two upper chambers of the heart quiver rather than beat efficiently.

And women have more episodes of hemorrhagic—or bleeding—strokes than men, who are more prone to a blocked blood supply that triggers the attack. That may also partly affect the way each sex experiences the illness, Morgenstern said, but it doesn't fully explain the dichotomy.

WHAT IS A STROKE?...

Strokes occur when a blood vessel that transports nutrients and oxygen to the brain either bursts or is blocked by a clot or atherosclerotic plaque. Either way, the area of the brain deprived of oxygen begins to die. And that, in turn, affects the part of the body that area controls.

Doctors have long known that the two sexes often show dissimilar signs of other cardiovascular problems, most notably heart attack.

Recently they've found that a woman is likely to be older than a man when she has her first stroke, and that the stroke is often more disabling and severe.

WOMEN SHOULD REDUCE RISKS...

Health professionals may not always recognize underlying conditions that can lead to a woman's stroke, according to some doctors. They may dismiss symptoms that might boost the risk of stroke in women.

Therefore, women should learn how best to reduce their risk of stroke and know when to ask for a thorough evaluation, experts believe.

For instance, it might be especially important for women to keep blood pressure under control, said Roquer. Other preventive measures include not smoking, avoiding obesity and not abusing alcohol and drugs, he says.

Rosabel Young, MD, is another stroke expert who sees certain gender differences in her stroke patients. "Generally women seem to have more embolic than thrombolic" stroke, said Young, a clinical assistant professor of neurology at UCLA's David Geffen School of Medicine.

Embolic strokes are caused by clots that start in the heart or the neck's carotid artery and move to the brain. Thrombotic strokes involve stationary clots in blood vessels.

"[Usually], embolic strokes are worse," Dr. Young added, "and have more complications."

For women, especially older women, heeding the physical symptoms they may experience is crucial. And they should try to reduce their cardiovascular risk factors by lowering blood cholesterol and quitting smoking, both Young and Roquer said.

ALSO: "If you have dizziness or panic attack symptoms and irregular heart rate, you should be checked out thoroughly for heart disease or stroke," Young added.

Dr. Morgenstern said that doctors should look for stroke in women complaining of unconventional symptoms because "time is of the essence" for effective treatments such as clot-busting drugs, which must be administered within the first few hours of symptom onset to be effective.

■

BEYOND THE SNIFFLES: ALLERGIES CAN TRIGGER VERY SURPRISING SYMPTOMS

Sources: **Thomas Brunoski, MD,** specialist in the treatment of medical problems and food and environmental allergies through the use of nutritional and preventive methods...*Bottom Line/Personal.*

Allergic reactions to pollen, mold, food and other substances affect the *entire* body—not just the nose or sinuses. The symptoms can be far more serious than sniffles and sneezes. Yet few people connect persistent illness to allergies.

CASE STUDY #1: SKIN RASH...

A young woman had been treated successfully for allergy-triggered skin rashes as well as sinus problems. She came back with head-to-toe eczema that had appeared after she moved into a new home.

Testing showed several allergies. The strongest was to dogs, yet none of her neighbors owned a dog.

SOLUTION: Although the new house had been professionally cleaned, urine stains from the previous owner's dog were embedded in the wood floor. After the stains were removed—part of the floor had to be replaced—her eczema vanished.

CASE STUDY #2: ASTHMA...

A nine-month-old child had severe asthma and eczema, which had not improved even after the doctor had prescribed an oral steroid.

Because this medication can stunt a child's growth and damage the immune system, the mother was understandably distraught.

I uncovered a powerful allergy to oranges. Yet the baby did not eat oranges or drink orange juice.

SOLUTION: I advised the mother to check around her home. She discovered the furniture polish she used contained orange fragrance. When she discarded the polish and removed all traces from the furniture, her son's symptoms cleared up.

CASE STUDY #3: CANKER SORES...

For years, a woman suffered from unpredictable and recurring canker sores. Despite a range of treatments, from medicated mouthwash to antibiotics, the sores persisted.

Since allergies can aggravate inflammation, I advised an allergy test. The results showed a reaction to dairy products.

SOLUTION: An analysis of her diet revealed that her on-and-off consumption of dairy products—ice cream in the summer—explained why the sores appeared sporadically. Avoiding dairy products completely has kept the sores away.

CASE STUDY #4: SINUS TROUBLE...

A man had no relief from recurrent sinus infections, even after many courses of antibiotics. Allergy tests revealed that he was allergic to pollen, dust and molds.

He followed instructions to remove these allergens from his environment—but still experienced symptoms.

SOLUTION: The environment is not the only source for molds. Diet may also be a supplier. I advised him to avoid products that are fermented, such as cheese, vinegar (he had to check salad dressings) and pickles (which might garnish a hamburger and be in tartar sauce and other dressings)...and to switch to a low-yeast bread, such as sourdough. His sinus problems cleared.

DIAGNOSING ALLERGIES...

It is estimated that 17% to 21% of us suffer from allergies. Pollution is thought to be the main cause. The first step in discovering an allergy trigger is testing. Skin tests, once the sole diagnostic tool, can yield false-positive or false-negative results.

Instead, I use a blood test called the amplified ELISA. This highly accurate test identifies a broad range of allergens. No one is ever allergic to just one substance. This blood test also measures the intensity of the individual's reaction to each trigger.

Once the trigger is discovered, the source might still be unclear. Additional detective work generally uncovers the source, as the four case studies illustrate.

OVERCOMING ALLERGIES...

Identifying an allergen and avoiding heavy exposure to it are only the first two steps.

Because it's impossible to avoid many common allergens, I also recommend *desensitization*. During this process, a person is exposed gradually to increasing amounts of an allergen. Allergy shots—an injectable "cocktail" composed of multiple allergens—are typically prescribed. However, they sometimes have disappointing results...and can cause swelling, redness and soreness.

MORE EFFECTIVE: Allergy drops, a concentrate of a specific allergen. Patients take a weekly dose, under the tongue, for about two years.

I retest for allergies after one year. By then, most patients show great improvement.

With consistent therapy, the individual will eventually be able to withstand exposure to a once-troublesome allergen with little or no reaction.

TO FIND A PRACTITIONER: American Academy of Environmental Medicine, 316-684-5500...*www.aaem.com.*

STAYING HEALTHY...

Follow these basic steps to build good health and minimize your risk of allergic reactions...

• *Eat a variety of foods.* Humans evolved as hunter-gatherers who sampled many foods. We still do best with this type of diet. Even a moderate allergy may intensify with the daily consumption of trigger foods. And alternating foods makes it easier to spot possible triggers if symptoms occur.

• *Avoid processed foods.* Processing removes nutrients. Additives, preservatives and dyes are common triggers of allergic symptoms. Eat lots of fresh vegetables and fruits. Use cold-pressed, extra-virgin olive oil when cooking and in salad dressing. It contains essential fatty acids.

• *Take nutritional supplements.* With heavy processing and soil deletion, food may not always provide essential nutrients. I RECOMMEND THE FOLLOWING DAILY SUPPLEMENTS TO MANY OF MY PATIENTS...

• Multivitamin/multimineral containing 50 milligrams (mg) or more of B-complex vitamins.

• Chelated calcium to keep bones strong, 1,200 mg.

• Magnesium, which aids in absorption of calcium, 600 to 750 mg.

• Folic acid, which reduces the blood level of homocysteine, an amino acid that is harmful to the heart, 800 micrograms (mcg).

The amount that is available in over-the-counter pills is limited. Your doctor can write a prescription if you need a higher dose.

• Vitamin C, an antioxidant, 1,000 mg. Take 500 mg twice daily.

• *Exercise regularly.* Try to fit in at least a one-hour workout three times a week, preferably a combination of some kind of aerobic exercise and strength training.

ALL ABOUT "SINUS" HEADACHES

Source: **Alan Hirsch, MD,** founder and neurological director of Smell & Taste Treatment and Research Foundation in Chicago. He is a neurologist and psychiatrist and author of *What Your Doctor May Not Tell You About Sinusitis.* Warner.

Chances are, you or someone you know has gone to the doctor complaining of nasal congestion and a throbbing pain near one eye, and been diagnosed with a sinus headache due to sinus infection—and been prescribed antibiotics.

There is also a very good chance that the doctor was flat-out wrong—and that the antibiotics were both uncalled for and ineffective.

In fact, true sinusitis is actually quite rare. In one study of more than 3,000 patients initially diagnosed with sinusitis, a careful examination found that only *eight* of them (three-tenths of 1%) had a sinus infection.

Why is this misdiagnosis so common? One reason is that people have seen so many decongestant commercials on television depicting the sinuses as sources of pain that they automatically assume any headache in these areas must be caused by sinus congestion.

In reality, such headaches may be caused by a number of conditions. To make things even more confusing, these other conditions frequently cause misleading nasal symptoms as well.

But if it's not sinusitis causing that headache or feeling of fullness around your eye, then what is ailing you? HERE ARE THE MOST LIKELY CULPRITS...

MIGRAINE...

Migraine headaches are common mimics of sinus headaches, especially when combined with allergies. Migraine symptoms often include stuffiness on one side of the face, runny nose and a feeling of fullness in the head. In one study, headache researchers carefully examined 47 patients with self-reported sinus headaches and found that 98% were actually suffering from some type of migraine.

At the same time, 87% of the group also reported having nasal symptoms—either stuffiness, a runny nose or both. These patients had already been treated at other clinics, and many had been prescribed oral antihistamines and corticosteroid nasal sprays, such as *flunisolide* (Nasalide), in an attempt to relieve the headache.

Meanwhile, their underlying migraines went untreated. Not surprisingly, two-thirds of the patients were dissatisfied with their initial treatment. On the other hand, when the patients were asked to treat their headaches with *sumatriptan* (Imitrex)—a migraine medication that targets receptors in the nerves and blood vessels of the head—two-thirds of them reported little or no pain two hours later.

If you have recurring headaches, especially on one side of the head, it's important that you be carefully evaluated for migraine—and rule out other problems that could be causing your pain.

If it turns out that you are suffering from migraines, a variety of effective medications are now available. To relieve the pain in mid-attack, the first-line treatment of choice is a group of drugs called triptans, which include sumatriptan, available as a nasal spray or oral medication, and the oral medications *rizatriptan* (Maxalt), *naratriptan* (Amerge), *almotriptan* (Axert), *eletriptan* (Relpax), *zolmitriptan* (Zomig) and *frovatriptan* (Frova). Talk to your doctor about these as well as nondrug migraine treatments, such as the supplements magnesium sulfate and riboflavin.

COMMON COLD...

There's no question that a cold can sometimes lead to a sinus infection by causing the nasal passages to swell until mucus stagnates in the sinuses and becomes a breeding ground for bacteria.

But many lingering colds are diagnosed as having turned into sinusitis when in fact they haven't.

REASON: One of the criteria for a possible sinus infection is a cold that lasts more than 10 days. Yet studies show that many colds last 10 days or longer and are still just colds.

RESULT: A quarter of a billion colds per year in the US alone that could potentially be misdiagnosed as sinusitis—and mistreated with antibiotics.

One study found that 85% of "sinusitis" patients who either did nothing or received a placebo improved on their own within a couple of weeks, after their colds (which is all they had) had run their course.

ALLERGIES...

The symptoms of allergic rhinitis (an allergy-related inflammation of the nasal passages) can often be confused with sinusitis, especially in someone who is suffering from both allergies and a migraine. These symptoms typically include nasal stuffiness and sneezing, thin, clear mucus, a dry cough and sometimes a headache.

HOW TO TELL THAT IT'S ALLERGIES AND NOT A SINUS INFECTION: Symptoms of true sinusitis include a thick (not thin) nasal discharge and a phlegm-producing (not dry) cough. Treatment with an antihistamine should help relieve the nasal symptoms of allergy, but further allergy testing—as well as treatment for a possible underlying migraine condition—may also be needed.

ARTERITIS...

If you're over age 60, any type of headache that you haven't experienced before needs to be carefully evaluated for *temporal arteritis*—an inflammation of the temporal artery that runs down the temple beside the eye that can lead to stroke or blindness. Symptoms include a throbbing pain, swelling and tenderness in the temple area. If arteritis is suspected, your doctor may want to do a biopsy of the cells in the artery wall to confirm the diagnosis. Treatment typically involves administering *prednisone*, a corticosteroid, for one to two years.

WHEN YOU DO HAVE SINUSITIS...

If you have these signs on a chronic basis—a stuffed-up nose... thick green or yellow nasal discharge...facial discomfort, which may include pressure or pain mostly on one side of the face...an ache in the teeth...halitosis (bad breath)...pain, pressure or a feeling of fullness in the ears—then you may be one of the rare few suffering from true sinusitis. To confirm a diagnosis of sinusitis, doctors will often order a CT scan, but be warned—70% of the population has some sort of sinus abnormality, such as sinus mucosal thickening, that will show up on a CT scan, and most of these abnormalities have nothing to do with any sinus symptoms. The only sure way to determine whether a sinus infection exists is to do a sinus puncture, in which mucus is removed from the maxillary sinus (the only sinus in which the procedure can be done) and evaluated.

If you do have a true sinus infection, oral antibiotics will *not* cure it, because they're not strong enough. Any sinus infection should be treated immediately with a course of intravenous (IV) antibiotics, administered in a hospital setting.

■

IS IT SINUSITIS?

Source: **Alan Hirsch, MD,** founder and neurological director of Smell & Taste Treatment and Research Foundation in Chicago. He is a neurologist and psychiatrist and author of *What Your Doctor May Not Tell You About Sinusitis.* Warner.

As many as 45 million cases of sinusitis are diagnosed by doctors each year—and about nine times out of 10, the diagnosis is wrong.

Sinusitis, also called a sinus infection, is a bacterial infection of the sinus linings. Infection causes these linings to swell and interferes with the normal drainage of mucus. This results in congestion, headache, reduced sense of smell and/or taste, tenderness around the eyes, cheeks, nose and/or forehead as well as other symptoms.

The majority of patients who think (or have been told) that they have sinusitis actually have other conditions—allergies, a cold or migraine headaches. Errors in diagnosing sinusitis are a leading cause of unnecessary treatments, including the use of antibiotics and even surgery.

CAUSES AND DIAGNOSIS...

Behind the face, there are many small sinus cavities—over the eyes, along and behind the nose, above the teeth, etc. The cavities have tiny holes (ostia) that drain into the nose. Anything that interferes with normal drainage causes mucus to accumulate. The mucus provides a rich medium for bacterial growth and infection.

Many people have anatomical abnormalities, such as a deviated septum, that inhibit drainage and make them vulnerable to sinusitis. Other causes include colds, allergies and other conditions that trigger congestion.

Most cases of sinusitis are acute, lasting one to two weeks, and get better on their own without medical treatment. Less often, sinusitis is chronic, lasting three months or more. Patients who get four or more cases of acute sinusitis annually also are considered to have the chronic form. Chronic sinusitis may clear up without treatment, but less often than the acute form.

Most people with sinusitis have a greenish nasal discharge, a fever of more than 100°F, swollen lymph nodes and tenderness over the sinuses.

The only sure way to diagnose sinusitis is with a sinus puncture. The patient is given a local anesthetic. A needle is guided through a nostril into a sinus cavity to extract mucus. The mucus is examined in a laboratory for signs of bacterial infection. Other sinusitis tests include CT and MRI scans, though these aren't as accurate as the sinus puncture.

TREATMENT AND PREVENTION...

Doctors routinely prescribe oral antibiotics to patients who appear to have sinusitis, but subjects in studies who are given no treatment recover just as quickly as those given antibiotics.

The only effective treatments for sinusitis are intravenous antibiotics given for three days to a week in the hospital...or surgery to restore normal drainage in the sinus cavities. Few patients need these treatments because true sinusitis is rare.

However, most patients can control sinus discomfort, regardless of the underlying cause, and lower the risk of infection by reducing or eliminating congestion. **BEST APPROACHES...**

• *Drink at least eight glasses of water daily.* It thins mucus in the sinuses and promotes normal drainage. This is especially important if you have a cold or allergy flare-up.

• *Don't take over-the-counter antihistamines or decongestants.* They dry mucus and impede normal drainage.

• *Ask your doctor about sumatriptan (Imitrex).* This medication, typically prescribed for migraines, can relieve sinusitus symptoms, postnasal drip, nasal congestion, a sense of fullness/pressure in the face, etc. The drug is effective in about 75% of cases.

• *Irrigate with a neti pot.* Available in natural-health stores, a neti pot looks like a small teapot. It is used to flush a saline solution through the nose, nasal passages and sinuses.

Flushing these areas once or twice daily when you're congested can improve drainage and reduce symptoms—or prevent sinusitis when you're suffering from a cold or allergies.

Mix about one-third teaspoon of salt and a pinch of baking soda in one cup of lukewarm water. Pour the solution into the neti pot.

Rotate and tip your head over a sink, and pour the solution into one nostril. Keep pouring until it flows out of the other nostril.

Spit out any fluid that enters the mouth. Then repeat on the other side.

■

REDUCED SENSE OF SMELL MAY SIGNAL LARGER PROBLEMS

Source: **Alan Hirsch, MD,** founder and neurological director of Smell & Taste Treatment and Research Foundation in Chicago. He is a neurologist and psychiatrist and author of *What Your Doctor May Not Tell You About Sinusitis.* Warner.

Half of all people over age 65 have a diminished sense of smell, called *hyposmia.* Although this condition often is a normal part of aging or a temporary symptom of a cold, it also can indicate a serious medical problem.

Head injury and neurological conditions, such as Alzheimer's disease, are associated with hyposmia. A loss of smell can be the first symptom of a tumor on the *hypothalamus* (a region of the forebrain that controls body temperature and appetite) or a nasal polyp.

Hyposmia also is linked to an underactive thyroid (hypothyroidism), which is diagnosed by a simple blood test and treated with a thyroid hormone replacement medication. Diminished sense of smell is an early symptom of some forms of breast cancer, as well.

Most patients—and even some doctors—don't realize that many medications can inhibit one's sense of smell.

MOST COMMON OFFENDERS: The cholesterol-lowering drug *rosuvastatin* (Crestor)...the antipsychotics *haloperidol* (Haldol) and *chlorpromazine* (Thorazine)...the antidepressant *nortriptyline* (Pamelor)...and the stimulant *methyl-phenidate* (Ritalin), taken for attention-deficit hyperactivity disorder (ADHD) and mild depression in older adults.

If a medication is to blame, a doctor often can alter the dosage or substitute a different medication.

DANGER: Without smell, the ability to savor food is greatly impaired. No longer able to smell or taste, people who have hyposmia often overeat and/or use too much salt on their food, unhealthful practices that can result in obesity and/or high blood pressure.

How to protect yourself...

DIAGNOSIS...

Test your sense of smell. Have your spouse or a friend prepare separate dishes of chocolate and vanilla ice cream. While blindfolded, taste a spoonful of each. If you can identify the flavors, chances are your olfactory system is functioning properly. Approximately 90% of what we perceive as taste really is smell.

If you are concerned about the results of your self-test, or think your sense of smell may be impaired, speak to your doctor about a "smell test."

During such a test, your doctor will probably ask you to close your eyes. He/she will then wave a strong-smelling object, such as an alcohol pad, about seven inches from your nose. If you can identify the odor, your sense of smell is most likely normal.

You also may receive an *olfactory threshold test*—a presentation of bottles that emit various odors, such as rose or chemicals, in different concentrations—to detect your smell acuity.

Also included is a smell identification test in which you are asked to identify different odors, such as soap, coffee and cloves.

IMPORTANT: Before visiting your doctor, list all the drugs you take. Write a brief description of any recent illnesses, including primary symptoms, and whether the condition worsens or improves at certain times. Also note whether you have any relatives who have hyposmia. In some people, the condition may have a genetic link.

If your primary doctor is unable to diagnose your problem, he may refer you to an ear, nose and throat specialist (otolaryngologist) if he suspects a nasal condition, such as nasal polyps or structural lesions obstructing airflow to the nose. If there are signs of a neurological problem, such as a brain tumor or multiple sclerosis, your doctor may refer you to a neurologist.

GOOD IDEA: If you determine that your sense of smell is impaired, get a "smell buddy," a person whom you trust to tell you whether you have foul-smelling breath or offensive odors in your home.

Make sure you have a working smoke detector and gas detector—as well as a carbon monoxide detector (even though this gas is odorless). All these products are available at hardware stores.

HOW TO IMPROVE YOUR SENSE OF SMELL...

Change your diet. Sense of smell and taste depends on proper functioning of the olfactory nerves and the *trigeminal nerve*. This nerve is stimulated when irritant molecules are inhaled through the nose. If your olfactory nerves have deteriorated due to aging, try "waking up" your trigeminal nerve.

SMART IDEA: Eat flavors that arouse the trigeminal nerve, including spearmint, horseradish, fresh onion, curries, hot chilis and cinnamon. Whip (aerate) your food, using a fork, food processor or blender, if possible, to arouse the odor-generating molecules.

Ask your doctor about taking *phosphatidylcholine*. This dietary supplement improves the sense of smell by raising the levels of the brain chemical *acetylcholine*, one of the neurotransmitters involved in the transmission of the olfactory impulse. Phosphatidylcholine is available in health-food stores.

TYPICAL DOSE: Nine grams per day taken in a divided dose at breakfast, lunch and dinner.

■

WHAT YOU CAN DO TO SAVE YOUR SIGHT

Source: **Gregory K. Harmon, MD,** associate professor of clinical ophthalmology at Weill Medical College of Cornell University and director of Glaucoma Service at New York Presbyterian Hospital, both in New York City. He is chairman and CEO of the Glaucoma Foundation, the nation's leading nonprofit organization promoting glaucoma research. *www.glaucomafoundation.org.*

Glaucoma is the second-leading cause of blindness in the US (after macular degeneration). It shouldn't be. Nearly all cases can be treated easily. The problem is that the most common form of glaucoma typically causes no symptoms until vision is impaired. At least half of glaucoma patients aren't diagnosed until they have suffered permanent vision damage. Most patients develop blind spots in their peripheral field of vision.

Continuing deterioration of the optic nerve can lead to blindness in one or both eyes. Damage occurs over years or decades—or, sometimes, within hours.

MAIN TYPES...

There are more than 40 subtypes of glaucoma. Most occur when fluids in the eye drain too slowly or stop draining. This happens when particles clog the sieve-like drainage system (trabecular meshwork) or when the drainage angle formed by the cornea and iris closes or is narrower than it should be. Buildup of fluid causes pressure within the eye to rise. Too much pressure can damage the optic nerve.

Main types of glaucoma...

• *Open-angle glaucoma* accounts for two-thirds of cases in the US. The fluid (*aqueous humor*) in the eye drains too slowly. Open-angle glaucoma progresses so slowly that many patients suffer substantial vision loss before they know there's a problem.

• *Angle-closure glaucoma* occurs when the drainage canal is blocked. Symptoms include severe pain, blurred vision, nausea and/or vomiting. People with these symptoms must get to an emergency room immediately. Acute angle-closure glaucoma can cause blindness within hours.

EARLY DETECTION...

The American Academy of Ophthalmology recommends that healthy adults get screened for glaucoma at least once in their 20s, twice in their 30s, every two to four years between the ages of 40 and 64, and every one to two years thereafter.

Those with risk factors for glaucoma—a family history... chronic conditions, such as diabetes or hypertension...a history of eye injuries or being farsighted—should get screened more often. African-Americans are much more likely than Caucasians to get glaucoma, and Asians have a higher risk for angle-closure glaucoma. People in these groups should ask their doctors about screening frequency.

To test for glaucoma, your doctor will probably perform these three exams...

• *Tonometry.* This simple procedure measures intraocular pressure. A reading higher than 23 mm/Hg means that a patient has an elevated risk of developing glaucoma.

- *Visual field test.* A computer generates dots of different sizes and brightness in different parts of the patient's visual field to detect blind spots.
- *Ophthalmoscopy.* The doctor uses an ophthalmoscope to examine the retina.

TREATMENT FOR OPEN-ANGLE GLAUCOMA...

Open-angle glaucoma often can be treated with medications, which can lower eye pressure by as much as 35%. That's frequently enough to stop the progression of the disease.

- *Hypotensive lipids* (Lumigan, Xalatan, Travatan) are the newest drugs. Usually given in drop form once a day, they accelerate the drainage of eye fluids.

SOME POSSIBLE SIDE EFFECTS: Temporary stinging or burning, eye redness, increased eyelash growth or darkening of the skin beneath the eyes.

About 10% of patients don't respond to these drugs and may require different medications, which can be used alone or in combination with hypotensive lipids.

- *Adrenergic agents* (Iopidine, Alphagan P), usually given in drop form two to three times daily, reduce the body's production of fluid in the eye.

POSSIBLE SIDE EFFECTS: Eye redness, itching, dizziness, dry mouth.

- *Beta-blockers,* such as *timolol,* usually given in drop or gel form once or twice daily, reduce eye fluids.

POSSIBLE SIDE EFFECTS: Slowed pulse, difficulty breathing, impotence, fatigue.

SURGERY...

If a patient doesn't achieve adequate lowering of pressure with drug treatment, surgery may be needed...

- *Laser surgery (argon laser trabeculoplasty),* performed on an outpatient basis, shrinks portions of the trabecular meshwork, which gives other parts of the network room to expand and makes it easier for fluids to drain. About 75% of patients who undergo laser surgery achieve an adequate lowering of eye pressure. However, the effects of laser surgery may decline over time.

BREAKTHROUGH: Selective laser trabeculoplasty causes little inflammation and no scarring. Patients can have repeat procedures to control eye pressure. With older lasers, patients could have the procedure only two or three times.

• *Traditional surgery (trabeculectomy),* performed in a hospital or outpatient clinic, is used when laser surgery isn't effective. The goal is to open a passageway in the white (sclera) of the eye. The surgeon goes through the hole to remove part of the trabecular meshwork and promote drainage. The procedure is successful in about 90% of cases, but it is more likely to cause scarring than laser procedures.

TREATMENT FOR ANGLE-CLOSURE GLAUCOMA...

Angle-closure glaucoma patients first are given eyedrops that reduce pressure quickly. Then patients undergo laser peripheral iridotomy, a surgical procedure that creates a hole in the iris to allow fluid drainage. Patients may need additional procedures to remove scar tissue and improve the drainage angle.

PREVENTION...

There is no proven way to prevent glaucoma, although a study found that patients with elevated eye pressure who took medicated drops were half as likely to develop glaucoma as those who didn't take them. Ask your doctor if preventive drops are right for you.

Lifestyle factors may help prevent glaucoma. BEST...

• *Exercise most days of the week.* It improves circulation and can slightly lower eye pressure. Some patients can reduce their medication once they start aerobic activities, such as brisk walking.

WARNING: Avoid head-down positions in yoga. They can increase eye pressure.

• *Eat nutritious foods.* Dark green, leafy vegetables, such as spinach and kale, are particularly beneficial.

• *Take a multivitamin/mineral supplement that contains zinc and antioxidants,* including vitamin C, vitamin E and carotenoids, such as lutein and zeaxanthine.

• *Don't smoke.* The nicotine in cigarettes may cause the veins in the eyes to constrict, inhibiting drainage.

■

THREE COMMON VIRUSES INCREASE RISK OF DEMENTIA

Sources: **Howard E. Gendelman, MD,** director, Center for Neurovirology and Neurodegenerative Disorders, University of Nebraska Medical Center, Omaha... **Larry Goldstein, MD,** professor of medicine and director of the stroke center, Duke University Medical Center, Durham, NC... *Stroke.*

Three fairly common viruses appear to increase the risk that elderly people will get dementia, according to a study. People with a history of infection with at least two of the viruses —two strains of herpes and a microbe called cytomegalovirus—were approximately twice as likely to show significant mental decline during the one-year study as those infected with one or none of the pathogens.

THE VIRUSES...

Herpes and cytomegalovirus are known to damage brain cells, so infection with either or both viruses could lead to the loss of neurons, and eventually dementia, according to the researchers.

In theory, drugs to treat existing infections or vaccines to prevent infections could prevent dementia.

THE INFLAMMATION CONNECTION...

Scientists are beginning to recognize that a variety of brain diseases, from Alzheimer's to Parkinson's, have at least some connection to inflammation.

In elderly patients, inflammation from a localized infection in another part of the body can undermine the integrity of the blood-brain barrier, allowing harmful molecules to pass into the brain that normally wouldn't be able to, according to Howard Gendelman, MD, director of the Center for Neurovirology and Neurodegenerative Disorders at the University of Nebraska Medical Center in Omaha.

This process can damage neurons and lead to dementia. It often does so in HIV patients, for example, he said.

Yet not all dementia results from infection, and not all infections lead to dementia. Genetics, nutrition and other factors likely affect a person's susceptibility to brain inflammation, Dr. Gendelman said.

THE STUDY...

In the study, Timo Strandberg, MD, of the University of Helsinki in Finland, and his colleagues followed up 383 elderly men and women with varying stages of blood vessel disease. More than 80% of the study participants had a history of heart disease and 37% had had at least one stroke.

THE RESEARCHERS LOOKED FOR SIGNS OF INFECTION WITH THREE COMMON VIRUSES: Herpes simplex 1, which causes cold sores...a related sexually transmitted virus, herpes simplex 2...and cytomegalovirus, which can be harmful to babies in the womb but typically causes no problems for healthy adults.

Blood tests revealed that 48 people had evidence, in the form of proteins called antibodies, of one or none of the viruses...229 had antibodies to two of the microbes...and 106 had signs of infection with all three viruses.

At the beginning of the study, 58 people (15%) had cognitive trouble on a standard psychological exam.

Subjects with antibodies to three viruses were 2.5 times more likely to fall into this group than people with fewer or no infections.

The greater the level of antibodies (that is, the greater the number of infections), the more severe the dementia.

During the following 12 months, 150 of the subjects lost ground on the cognitive test. Again, history of infection was strongly linked to the likelihood of mental decline.

CAUTION URGED...

Larry Goldstein, MD, director of the Duke University Stroke Center and a spokesman for the American Stroke Association, cautions that the Finnish findings may not translate to other groups of people. Not only did all the subjects have some form of vessel disease, but Finland is far more ethnically homogenous than the United States.

The study "is not applicable to the general population. It's limited to that narrow group of folks," Dr. Goldstein said.

For more on dementia, visit the National Library of Medicine at *www.nlm.nih.gov* or the Alzheimer's Association at *www.alz.org*.

■

SPOT AND TREAT SHINGLES QUICKLY

Source: **Leon Kircik, MD,** medical director, Physicians Skin Care and Dermato-
logic Research, PLLC, Louisville, KY. He is also a consulting physician at Jewish
Hospital, Louisville, and Staten Island University Hospital, New York City.

Shingles is a painful nerve ailment caused by the reactiva-
tion of the chicken pox virus in adulthood. One out of every
five Americans will have shingles at some point in his/her life.

While the disease can occur at any age, it usually strikes
after age 50 and is most common among people ages 65 to 80.
Shingles rarely occurs more than once and typically lasts a
week to 10 days. But if not treated promptly with medication,
that single episode can result in painful nerve damage that
persists for years.

WHAT CAUSES SHINGLES?...

To get shingles, you must already have been exposed to the
chicken pox virus earlier in life.

After someone comes down with chicken pox, typically as a
child, the virus that caused it—a type of herpes virus known
as varicella-zoster virus (VZV) or herpes zoster—retreats to
nerve cells along the spinal cord, where it remains for life.

When immunity to VZV declines, either due to age or because
the immune system has been weakened by a disease (such as
cancer or AIDS) or medication (such as chemotherapy), the virus can suddenly flare up again as shingles.

SYMPTOMS TO WATCH FOR...

One of the unique aspects of shingles is that it occurs only
on one side of the body, along the affected nerve. The first
signs tend to be an unusual tingling, burning or itching sensation or an abnormal sensitivity along one arm, leg or cheek,
sometimes accompanied by flu-like symptoms. This indicates
that the virus has become active in the nerve root. Within a
few days—the time it takes for the virus to reach the skin—a
rash of painful, fluid-filled blisters develops in the area where
the nerve sensations occurred.

Left untreated, the blisters usually dry up on their own in
seven to 10 days, while prompt drug treatment can shorten
the episode to three or four days. Once the rash clears up,

however, 20% of shingles patients are left with ongoing nerve pain in the affected area that can last for months or even years—a condition called post-herpetic neuralgia. In the most severe cases, even the slightest touch causes excruciating pain to such an extent that normal activities become impossible.

VERY IMPORTANT: The best possible way to prevent post-herpetic neuralgia is to take antiviral medication within 72 hours of the first signs of tingling, burning or itching—before any blisters appear. (Just as with a herpes-related cold sore, medicine is applied at the first sign of tingling, before the sore actually appears.) Once the virus has reached the skin—in 48 to 72 hours—it's too late for the medication to have any preventive effect.

OTHER DANGERS OF SHINGLES: Shingles sometimes affects a nerve supplying the face. When this happens, the virus can spread to the eye or ear, leading to blindness or deafness if it's not treated quickly. Until they've dried up, the blisters are contagious, and direct contact with them could spread chicken pox (not shingles) to someone who has never had chicken pox.

If you have fresh shingles blisters, be especially careful not to get near a child who hasn't had chicken pox, anyone with a compromised immune system or a pregnant woman (whose fetus could be at risk if she catches chicken pox).

DIAGNOSING AND TREATING SHINGLES...

If you feel a strange sensation that you suspect may be shingles, your best bet is to see a dermatologist at once. Unless your primary care doctor is familiar with shingles, diagnosing the early signs, before the rash appears, can be difficult. The rash itself can also be misleading, since it may resemble herpes simplex or contact dermatitis. A trained dermatologist will be able to spot the symptoms of shingles immediately and confirm the diagnosis with a viral culture.

Once diagnosed, the shingles patient is immediately started on a seven- to 10-day course of the antiviral drug *acyclovir* (Zovirax)—taken five times a day—or *valacyclovir* (Valtrex) or *famciclovir* (Famvir), both of which are taken twice a day. As mentioned above, the earlier the antiviral drugs are given, the more effective they will be. To prevent long-term complications, they should be started no later than 72 hours after the first signs of shingles appear.

Additional treatments may include topical antibiotics, such as Bactroban ointment, to prevent infection, and topical steroids, such as hydrocortisone, to help dry up the blisters and reduce painful inflammation. The infected area must also be kept clean as an additional safeguard against secondary infections.

In severe cases, such as in those who have weak immune systems, shingles can cover the entire body or spread internally. In both of these cases, the patient may need to be hospitalized and given acyclovir intravenously. If the eye or ear becomes involved, then the patient will need to be referred to an eye or ear specialist for appropriate treatment. If the patient develops post-herpetic neuralgia, appropriate pain management will also be required.

■

DON'T IGNORE SPINAL PROBLEMS

Source: **Harry Herkowitz, MD,** chairman of orthopaedic surgery and director, section of spine surgery, William Beaumont Hospital, Royal Oak, MI.

M any people ignore minor aches and pains. Well, that isn't always the wisest thing to do. Some things should not be ignored, because they're dangerous.

Spinal stenosis is high on the list of diseases that cause great discomfort and that people do nothing about. Estimates are that some 400,000 Americans over the age of 60 have symptoms of spinal stenosis, and many of them don't even know what it is or that they have it.

SPINAL STENOSIS DEFINED...

Spinal stenosis is a narrowing of the spinal canal caused by a number of factors, including osteoarthritis of the spine, spinal damage from a previous fall, being born with a narrow spinal canal, and wear and tear on the vertebrae and joints that can come with aging. Additionally, lifestyle issues, such as being overweight, lack of exercise, poor general health and smoking, can also cause stenosis.

The narrowing eventually starts to pinch the spinal cord and nerves, and the result is pain. Stenosis nearly always causes pain in the lumbar (lower part) of the spine, but it can create pain in the buttocks and legs as well. Pain generally kicks in as the person stands up and starts to move about. The legs often feel tired and cramped as well. As the disease progresses, pain will make walking and moving increasingly difficult—even standing up straight can be uncomfortable because an erect posture compresses the spinal canal.

DIAGNOSIS...

According to Harry Herkowitz, MD, chairman of orthopaedic surgery and director of the section of spine surgery at William Beaumont Hospital in Royal Oak, Michigan, stenosis is sometimes confused with other conditions, among them arthritis, diabetic neuropathy (nerve damage) and vascular claudication, which is pain from impaired circulation in the lower legs. Hence, getting a proper diagnosis is extremely important to ensure effective treatment.

To diagnose spinal stenosis, the doctor usually requests magnetic resonance imaging (MRI), a computed axial tomography (CAT) scan or a myelogram (an X-ray taken after fluid is injected into the spinal canal).

TREATMENT...

The first line of treatment, said Dr. Herkowitz, is short-term restriction of activity followed by physical therapy to strengthen the muscles in the back, along with an activity that does not cause discomfort, such as riding on a stationary bike. Other recommendations for treatment include anti-inflammatory agents such as aspirin and ibuprofen, weight loss and the cessation of smoking.

HELPFUL: You can find relief by lying down and drawing your knees to your chest or by assuming the fetal position. Any position that can stretch out the spine reduces the compression on the nerves. Alternate applications of hot and cold compresses, called contrast therapy, may provide not only temporary relief, but reduce inflammation and slow the disease progress.

If exercise and anti-inflammatory medications are not effective, the next line of defense is an epidural—injections of cortisone into the epidural space in the spine. An epidural successfully relieves pain in about half of patients. Not only does an epidural decrease inflammation, doctors believe it may also flush out some of the inflammatory proteins in the area. Dr. Herkowitz said that patients may need more than one injection and that it is acceptable to have up to three over a six-month period.

THE PROCEDURE...

Getting an epidural isn't something you do in your local doctor's office. You must use a doctor who is qualified to administer epidurals, such as an anesthesiologist, radiologist, neurologist, physiatrist (a doctor who specializes in treating problems of the musculoskeletal system) or an orthopedic surgeon.

If you are taking aspirin or any other blood-thinning drugs, discuss this with your doctor ahead of time because you will probably need to stop taking them for a period around the time the epidural is performed to decrease the possibility of bleeding. Be sure that you are aware of the risks associated with this procedure.

Although complications are rare, 2% to 3% of patients experience a bad headache. Other complications are much less likely—less than 1% of patients experience nerve injury, infection, meningitis and anaphylaxis. Most problems come from inferior techniques in administering the epidural. Pain associated with the procedure is well controlled at the injection site, but muscle cramping may develop.

LAST RESORT—SURGERY...

The last alternative in the treatment process is a surgery known as laminectomy. The surgeon removes a portion of bone over the nerve root and also may trim part of any facet joints (small stabilizing joints between and behind the vertebrae) that are compressing the nerves. The goal is to give the spinal nerves more room. The surgery is successful for about 80% of patients, said Dr. Herkowitz. While surgery can cure a specific area of stenosis, there is still about a 10% chance that the patient will go on to develop stenosis in another area of the spine, which could require additional surgery. Risks include infection, a tear in the membrane that covers the spinal cord at the site of the surgery, bleeding, a blood clot in a leg vein, decreased intestinal function and neurologic deterioration, although these appear to be rare. The surgery should be performed by someone who is highly experienced in back surgery.

Although Dr. Herkowitz said there is nothing you can do to prevent spinal stenosis, there are many ways to treat it and to make yourself more comfortable. No matter what your age, you can and should seek treatment. Patients well into their 80s have benefited from laminectomy surgery. "Getting old" is never an excuse for not getting the proper medical care.

■

HOW SIMPLE SPRAINS CAN LEAD TO ARTHRITIS

Sources: **Victor Valderrabano, MD,** orthopedic physician and researcher, University of Basel, Switzerland, and Human Performance Laboratory, University of Calgary, Canada...**Stuart Miller, MD,** orthopedic surgeon, Union Memorial Hospital, Baltimore...American Orthopaedic Foot and Ankle Society meeting, Washington, DC.

Ankle sprains seem to boost the risk of developing painful osteoarthritis in the joint, research suggests.

This finding indicates that intensive rehabilitation is needed after chronic ankle instability or injury to help ward off the degenerative joint disease, say researchers.

For years, experts have known that arthritis in the ankle often occurs after a fracture in that joint, but there's been debate whether recurrent ankle sprains or instability—without a fracture—can lead to arthritis. The latest research says that it can, although not everyone agrees.

Swiss researchers evaluated 268 patients who had ankle arthritis. Of these, 83% had experienced a fracture in the past and 18% had chronic ankle instability with recurrent sprains but no fractures. In patients who experienced fractures, it took an average of 21 years from the time of injury to develop arthritis...among those with ankle injuries without a fracture, arthritis developed 22 years later.

This study is not the first to suggest the sprain-and-arthritis link, according to lead researcher Victor Valderrabano, MD, of the orthopedic department of the University of Basel.

Dr. Valderrabano said arthritis may develop after an ankle sprain because the weight from walking and other movements continues to stress the vulnerable joint.

Up to 40% of patients who have ankle injuries experience chronic instability in the joint, the authors said, and up to 80% of those people eventually will develop arthritis in the ankle.

However, not everyone agrees that the link between ankle sprains and arthritis is so clear-cut. "People have looked at this many times in the past and it has not held up to scientific scrutiny," said Stuart Miller, MD, an orthopedic surgeon at Union Memorial Hospital in Baltimore. Experts suspect a connection but have no definitive proof, he added.

Dr. Miller and the Swiss researchers agreed on one point— anyone who experiences recurrent ankle sprains needs an intensive rehabilitation program of physical therapy to strengthen muscles to become more immune to injury.

Osteoarthritis is characterized by the breakdown of the joint's cartilage. This loss of cartilage causes bones to rub against each other, causing pain and loss of movement, according to the Arthritis Foundation.

■

WARNING: BRUISES MAY BE A SIGN OF SOMETHING SERIOUS

Source: **Jerome Z. Litt, MD,** assistant clinical professor of dermatology, Case Western Reserve University School of Medicine, Cleveland. He is author of *Your Skin from A to Z*. Barricade.

Most bruises are just evidence of an active life—but if you get a bruise and it doesn't go away or you keep getting bruises, it could be a sign of a dangerous medical condition. **HERE'S WHAT YOU NEED TO KNOW...**

COMMON CAUSES...

When you fall or bump into something, small blood vessels (capillaries) near the skin's surface are broken.

Blood leaks out of the damaged vessels and seeps into adjoining tissues, leaving a discolored area.

Most bruises are initially bluish-black. Over a period of days, the blood pigment hemogloblin breaks down and triggers the release of bile pigments that cause bruises to change colors. The bruise gradually disappears as your body reabsorbs the blood and other fluids.

Some people bruise more easily than others. Women generally get more bruises than men because their skin is thinner —the hormone estrogen softens blood vessels and reduces the strength of collagen.

You're also more likely to bruise as you get older. These bruises, called Bateman's purpura, usually appear on the backs of the hands and the outer forearms. **REASONS...**

• *Capillaries* get thinner and weaker with age.

• *The protective fatty layer* in skin gets thinner and thus provides less protection.

• *Lifelong sun exposure* weakens collagen and other elastic tissues. This makes the blood vessels near the surface of the skin more vulnerable.

DRUG SIDE EFFECTS...

One adult aspirin (325 milligrams [mg]) can diminish the blood's ability to clot for up to six days—as well as increase your risk of bruises.

Other blood-thinning medications that cause bruising include *warfarin* (Coumadin) and *clopidogrel* (Plavix). Some dietary supplements, such as ginkgo biloba and garlic, also have blood-thinning effects.

SIGN OF DISEASE...

Bruises that appear even though you haven't been injured ...that are large or painful...or that are accompanied by bleeding elsewhere in the body may be a sign of leukemia or other blood disorders.

Frequent bruising also can be due to viral infections, such as herpes, measles, Epstein-Barr and HIV.

To diagnose the causes of bruising, your doctor may check blood platelet levels or the time it takes for blood to clot. You might need a bone marrow biopsy to check for leukemia or other blood disorders.

BRUISING Rx...

To prevent and heal common, everyday bruises...

• *Apply a cold pack or ice* wrapped in a washcloth as soon as possible after the injury. Hold for 20 minutes. Repeat several times. Cold constricts blood vessels, shortens clotting time and can reduce blood leakage from capillaries.

• *Elevate the injured area higher than your heart.* The longer you can do this, the better. It reduces blood flow to the injury.

• *Take vitamin C.* Vitamin C makes capillaries less fragile. Extra vitamin C is particularly important if you're taking aspirin or corticosteroids, drugs that can strip vitamin C from the body. The amount in a multisupplement, typically 60 to 100 mg, usually is adequate.

BONUS: Most multisupplements also contain zinc, a mineral that may reduce capillary leakage.

■

FOOD POISONING SELF-DEFENSE

Source: **Ewen Todd, PhD,** director, National Food Safety and Toxicology Center, Michigan State University, East Lansing. He previously headed the Contaminated Foods Section of the Health Protection Branch of the Canadian government.

There are an estimated 76 million cases of foodborne illness in the US each year. Many victims think they have contracted a "stomach flu" and never realize that food was actually to blame.

Most foodborne illnesses cause a day or two of nausea, diarrhea, abdominal cramping and, sometimes, vomiting. But in the US, 325,000 cases a year are severe enough to lead to hospitalization and about 5,200 are fatal, according to the Centers for Disease Control and Prevention. Foodborne illnesses are particularly dangerous for children under age five, adults over age 70, pregnant women and people with weakened immune systems.

Reduce your odds of infection by thoroughly cooking meats and setting your refrigerator to just above freezing for storing foods such as deli meat, pâté and smoked fish. Consume or freeze these foods within four or five days of purchase.

If you think you have food poisoning, drink lots of water and get plenty of rest.

CAUTION: Don't use antidiarrheal medications—they may slow the elimination of bacteria from your system.

Foodborne illness often improves within 48 hours. Call your doctor if you feel ill for longer than two or three days or if blood appears in your stool.

■

EATING DISORDERS ARE NOT JUST FOR TEENS ANYMORE

Source: **Shari Lusskin, MD,** reproductive psychiatrist and associate professor, New York University Medical Center, New York City.

Eating disorders such as anorexia or bulimia, which once affected mostly teenage girls, are a problem for a growing number of baby-boomer women.

Anorexia is characterized by weight loss due to excessive or compulsive dieting, often coupled with self-induced vomiting and chronic laxative use. Bulimia is defined as excessive binge eating, followed by purging or vomiting, and frequently, using laxatives.

Because the trend is so new, experts say there are no reliable studies to document how many women have eating disorders.

NEW FORM OF DISORDERS...

A relatively new expression of eating disorders is what some experts are calling "anorexercise," and it's attracting a substantial number of older women. They calculate every calorie consumed, and devise a workout designed to burn those exact number of calories—generally within 12 hours or less after eating.

"Some women will get up at 5 am to run, just to burn off what they ate the night before. And they can go to some very unhealthy extremes in using exercise to control their weight," said reproductive psychiatrist Shari Lusskin, MD, an associate professor at New York University School of Medicine.

HORMONAL CONNECTION?...

Although the causes of eating disorders are not fully understood, some experts believe hormones may play a role, particularly since the number of women affected far outweighs the number of men. According to the National Institutes of Mental Health, some 7 million American girls and women battle eating disorders, compared with 1 million boys and men.

And like the hormone fluctuations that occur during puberty —when young women are at risk for eating disorders—hormonal changes take place during perimenopause, when older women appear vulnerable as well.

Sometimes, undiagnosed depression is to blame, Dr. Lusskin said. "Because eating and depression can be so intimately entwined, it's likely that at least some older women with an eating disorder are really suffering from an undiagnosed depression, with a basic thread of unhappiness that ran through their lives for a long time and probably didn't come to the forefront until they hit middle age," she said.

The good news is that older women generally respond to treatment for eating disorders faster than younger women, and they are generally more motivated to seek help.

Treatment for all age groups includes counseling, medication, and, for older women, having a spouse involved in treatment.

Most important, according to many experts, is to join a support group. Studies show that sharing feelings with others facing a similar problem plays a major role in helping women of all ages overcome eating disorders.

WHAT ARE THE SYMPTOMS OF EATING DISORDERS?...

The National Institutes of Health (NIH) offers this explanation of different types of eating disorders and their symptoms...

• *Anorexia nervosa.* People who have anorexia develop unusual eating habits, such as avoiding meals, picking out a few foods and eating them in small amounts, weighing their food and counting the calories of everything they eat. They may also exercise excessively.

• *Bulimia nervosa.* People who have bulimia eat an excessive amount of food in a single episode and almost immediately make themselves vomit or use laxatives or diuretics to get rid of the food in their bodies. This behavior is referred to as the "binge/

purge" cycle. Like people who have anorexia, people who have bulimia also may have an intense fear of gaining weight.

• *Binge-eating disorder.* People who have this recently recognized disorder have frequent episodes of compulsive overeating, but unlike those with bulimia, they do not purge their bodies of food. During these food binges, they often eat alone and very quickly, regardless of whether they feel hungry or full. They often feel shame or guilt over their actions. Unlike anorexia and bulimia, binge-eating disorder occurs almost as often in men as in women.

To learn more about eating disorders, visit the National Eating Disorders Association at *www.nationaleatingdisorders.org.*

■